# B. JAIN'S
# GUIDE
## —— TO ——
# HOMEOPATHIC FAMILY KIT

### B. Jain's

# GUIDE
## to
# HOMEOPATHIC
# FAMILY KIT

*Includes*
- *Selection & Administration of Remedies*
- *Repetition of Doses* • *Precautions*

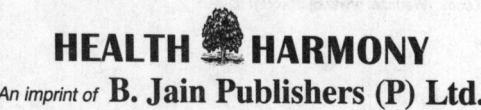

**HEALTH HARMONY**
*An imprint of* **B. Jain Publishers (P) Ltd.**
USA — EUROPE — INDIA

**B JAIN'S GUIDE TO HOMEOPATHIC FAMILY KIT**

First Edition: 1995
8th Impression: 2014

All rights reserved. No part of this book may be reproduced, stored in a retrieval system or transmitted, in any form or by any means, mechanical, photocopying, recording or otherwise, without any prior written permission of the publisher.

© with the publisher

Published by Kuldeep Jain for
**B. JAIN PUBLISHERS (P) LTD.**
1921/10, Chuna Mandi, Paharganj, New Delhi 110 055 (INDIA)
Tel.: +91-11-4567 1000   Fax: +91-11-4567 1010
Email: info@bjain.com   Website: **www.bjain.com**

Printed in India by
**JJ Imprints**

ISBN: 978-81-319-0104-5

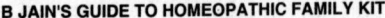

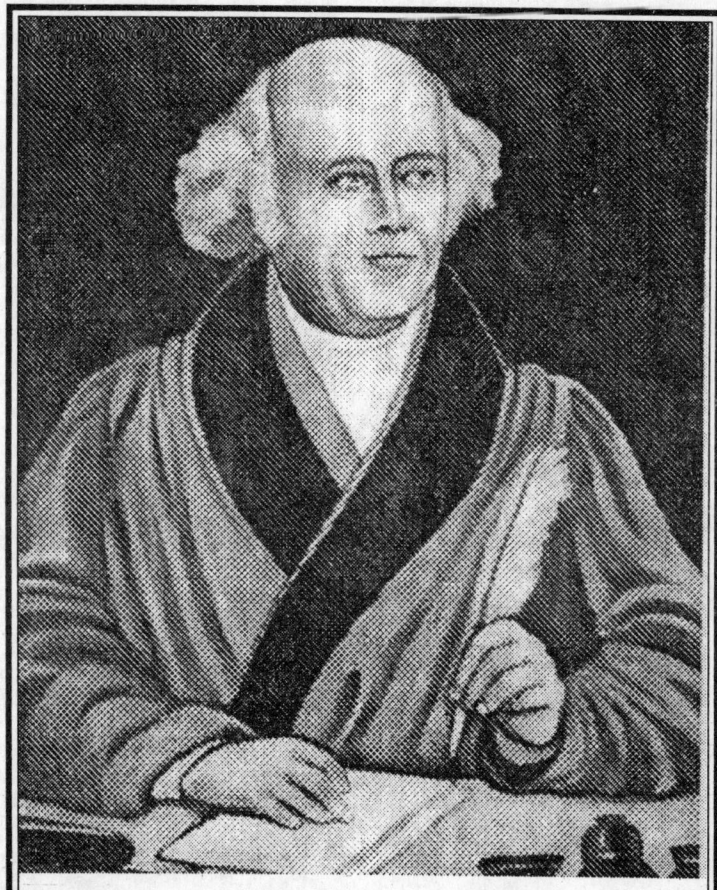

Dr. Samuel Hahnemann, 1755 to 1843

The development of his ideas on the new system of homoeopathy.

# CONTENTS

1. Publisher's note ................................................................. 3
2. The Goal ............................................................................ 5
3. Homoeopathy and Hahnemann ..................................... 7
4. Principles of Homoeopathy ............................................ 9
5. List of Remedies ............................................................. 11
6. Selection of Remedy ...................................................... 13
7. Administration of Remedies & repetition of Doses ............................................................. 15
8. Precautions ..................................................................... 17
9. Common Ailments and their Remedies ...................... 19
10. The Leading Indications of the recommended Remedies ............................................... 117
11. Books Recommended for Further Studies ................ 167

# 1 | PUBLISHER'S NOTE

This book is being offered to the general public with the honest intention of guiding the layman in the homoeopathic self-treatment or home treatment of common diseases not of a serious nature. This point the readers are urged to bear in mind.

The remedies indicated in the book have been prescribed on the basis of tips given by the stalwarts of homoeopathy, past and present. Authentic materials have also been collected from different sources and incorporated in this book.

The potency recommended here for each drug is 30. Only on gaining some good result with this potency can one go higher to 200 potency in case of illnesses of prolonged nature.

The final tip is — consult the physician in case of any difficulty.

**Dr. P.N. Jain**

# 2 | THE GOAL

None of us can deny that in today's overbusy life of ours we lack in one or the other of the two things which are of utmost importance, i.e., money and time. Obviously, many of us are earning handsomely and have got sufficient money to spend on health, yet no time to go to a doctor every now and then for our common ailments. On the other hand, in majority of the cases we may have sufficient time to visit the doctors but are unable to pay the treatment charges !

So, the objective of preparing this small book to supplement the vast ocean of homoeopathic literature is to introduce the **Homoeopathic System of Medicine** to every household by presenting a handy **Family Kit** which contains a repertory of 40 important homoeopathic remedies, and a few mother tinctures ($\phi$) and Mullein Oil. The remedies recommended here can be used by every literate member of the society without any harmful side-effects in the patient. It is hoped that the honourable members of the society will derive maximum benefit out of this small book by using the recommended remedies with utmost confidence in all circumstances, and they will be interested to procure further reading material to add to their knowledge.

# 3 | HOMOEOPATHY AND HAHNEMANN

The word Homoeopathy is a derivation from two Greek words, i.e., *"Homoios"* which means *"similar"* and *"pathos"* meaning *"disease"*. This system of medicine was enunciated by a German doctor, Samuel Christian Frederick Hahnemann, some 200 years ago. It is based on the natural law of cure, known as *similia similibus curantur* or "let likes be treated by likes". Dr. Hahnemann was born in Meissen on 10th April, 1755, and did his Doctorate in Medicine from Leipzig University at Erlanger in 1779 at the age of 24. He was a kind-hearted man and had great faith in the mercy of God.

During the days of Hahnemann the practice of medicine was a pretty crude affair, involving bleeding, purging and blistering, and was based on the speculative principles of orthodox medicine founded by Hippocrates. Disillusioned by this miserable condition of both the practice of medicine and the patients, he bade good-bye to his practice and decided to earn his living by translating medical books from one language to another. During this time around in the year 1790, he came across Cullen's explanation in his materia medica about *Cinchona* (a Peruvian bark) that it has the properties of curing Ague (malarial fever) because of its bitterness. Not satisfied, Dr. Hahnemann decided to verify the truth. He made a decoction of *Cinchona* and started taking its doses at frequent intervals. To his great astonishment, one day, all the characteristic symptoms of malarial fever appeared in him — *chill, heat* and *sweat*. Having confirmed the identical effects of *Cinchona* and other drug substances on his family members too, he concluded that a drug which is capable of producing disease like symptoms in a healthy person, can only prove curative in a patient if the patient has a similarity of symptoms which are produced by a deug in a healthy persons. This is what he called the *"Law of Similars", i.e., "Similia Similibus Curantur"* or *"let likes be treated by likes"*. The basic principles of Homoeopathy are enumerated in his book, "Organon of Medicine."

# 4 PRINCIPLES OF HOMOEOPATHY

The basic principles of Homoeopathy are as under :

1. **Law of Similars :** According to this law, the diseases should be treated by the remedies which have the properties of producing similar symptoms in a healthy person which are observed in the sickness of a patient..

2. **Doctrine of using Proved Remedies :** According to this law, only those remedies should be used for curative purposes which have been proved on healthy persons and their action is known to the physician.

3. **Doctrine of Single Remedy :** According to this law, only a single remedy should be used at one time so that it can manifest its pure action.

4. **Doctrine of Minimum Dose :** According to this law, the Homoeopathic remedies should be given in minute doses to avoid aggravation of symptoms in the patient and to bring about brilliant cures.

5. **Doctrine of Potentisation :** According to this principle, the homoeopathic medicines are potentised in dilutions and triturations as per the methods laid down in the homoeopathic pharmacopaeia. The potentised dilutions and triturations are marked with the symbols X or C for decimal or centesimal scales respectively. They are prepared in potencies from 1x to CMM/DMM and higher, but the most commonly used potencies are 3c, 3x, 6c, 6x, 12c, 12x, 30c, 30x, 200c, 200x, 1M, 10M, 50M, CM and DM. In the text all remedies have been recommended in the 30th potency, which is considered safe and mostly used.

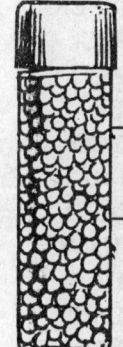

# 5 LIST OF REMEDIES

## (IN PILLS WITH 30 POTENCY)

| PHIAL NO. | NAME | ABBREVIATION |
|---|---|---|
| 1. | ACONITUM NAPELLUS | ACON. |
| 2. | AETHUSA CYNAPIUM | AETH-C. |
| 3. | ALLIUM CEPA | ALL-C. |
| 4. | ALOE SOCOTRINA | ALOES |
| 5. | ANTIMONIUM TARTARICUM | ANT-T. |
| 6. | APIS MELLIFICA | APIS |
| 7. | ARNICA MONTANA | ARN. |
| 8. | ARSENICUM ALBUM | ARS. |
| 9. | BELLADONNA | BELL. |
| 10. | BORAX | BOR. |
| 11. | BRYONIA ALBA | BRY. |
| 12. | CALCAREA PHOSPHORICA | CALC-P. |
| 13. | CANTHARIS | CANTH. |
| 14. | CARBO VEGETABILIS | CARB-V. |
| 15. | CHAMOMILLA | CHAM. |
| 16. | COCCULUS INDICUS | COCC. |
| 17. | COLOCYNTHIS | COLO. |
| 18. | CUPRUM METALLICUM | CUPR. |
| 19. | EUPHRASIA OFFICINALIS | EUPHR. |
| 20. | FERRUM PHOSPHORICUM | FERR-P. |
| 21. | GELSEMIUM | GELS. |

| | | |
|---|---|---|
| 22. | GLONOINE | GLON. |
| 23. | HEPAR SULPHUR | HEP. |
| 24. | HYPERICUM PERFORATUM | HYPER. |
| 25. | IPECACUANHA | IPEC. |
| 26. | LACHESIS | LACH. |
| 27. | LEDUM PALUSTRE | LED. |
| 28. | LYCOPODIUM CLAVATUM | LYCO. |
| 29. | MAGNESIA PHOSPHORICA | MAG-P. |
| 30. | MERCURIUS SOLUBILIS | MERC. |
| 31. | NUX VOMICA | NUX-V. |
| 32. | PHOSPHORUS | PHOS. |
| 33. | PLANTAGO MAJOR | PLANT. |
| 34. | PULSATILLA | PULS. |
| 35. | RHUS TOXICODENDRON | RHUS-T. |
| 36. | RUTA GRAVEOLENS | RUTA |
| 37. | SPIGELIA | SPIG. |
| 38. | SPONGIA TOSTA | SPONG. |
| 39. | SULPHUR | SULPH. |
| 40. | VERATRUM ALBUM | VERAT. |

**MOTHER TINCTURES & MULLEIN OIL**

| | |
|---|---|
| 41. | CALENDULA |
| 42. | CANTHARIS |
| 43. | PLANTAGO MAJOR |
| 44. | MULLEIN OIL |

# 6    SELECTION OF REMEDY

While selecting a remedy for a particular patient, it should always be borne in mind that the basic principle of homoeopathy is based on the Law of Similars. Hence the selection of remedy should not be made in the name of a disease, but only on the basis of the symptoms exhibited by the patient. In the text, such symptoms (as different from the disease) have been given under each ailment and the remedies indicated against them.

# 7 | ADMINISTRATION OF REMEDIES & REPETITION OF DOSES

The remedies can be administered both orally and locally. For oral use the kit contains 40 phials of leading homoeopathic remedies in globules (pills) No. 30. These phials have been numbered from 1 to 40 for easy handling. These numbers have also been put within brackets along with the indicated remedies given under common ailments to avoid any confusion. For local application we have **Calendula** (φ), **Cantharis** (φ), **Plantago major** (φ) and **Mullein oil** (φ). The applicability of these tinctures have been indicated in the treatment of some of the **common ailments, injuries,** etc.

Now diverting back to useS of oral remedies in their globul form, it may be noted that 1 globule makes a sufficient dose for an infant, 2 globules for a child and 3 globules for an adult. These globules should be given or taken dry on the tongue in a clean piece of paper, or dissolved on a clean spoonful of water. In very acute cases the doses can be administered at an interval of 15 to 30 minutes till the severe symptoms abate. Thereafter, the interval should be lengthened from an hour to 3-4 hours. Here, always keep in mind that, if a given remedy does not show a favourable response after 2-3 doses, or if the condition of your patient becomes worse, the doctor may be called in immediately or the patient should be rushed to a hospital. Till seeking appropriate medical aid the patient may be given one of the indicated remedies stocked in the family kit.

# 8 | SOME IMPORTANT INDICATIONS

1. Do not give or take any medicine unless you find a good deal of similarity between the symptoms of the patient and the remedy.
2. Do not give more than one medicine at a time.
3. Do not repeat a remedy too often, unless it be in exceptional circumstances. Stop the remedy as soon as the condition worsens.
4. Protect the **"Family Kit"** and other homoeopathic remedies from Camphor, strong perfumes, cosmetics and direct sunshine.
5. Drugs of any other kind, raw onions, garlic, asafoetida (*heeng*), coffee, peppermint, highly spiced food, beer and other alcoholic beverages should not be taken during homoeopathic treatment.
6. Do not use *Arsenicum album* during an acute stage of a cold or pneumonia.
7. Do not use *Apis mellifica* before and after *Rhus toxicodendron* as these are inimical to each other.
8. Do not use *Sulphur* before *Lycopodium*.
9. Do not use *Sulphur* in frequent doses and at night. It should always be administered in the morning, except in case of sleeplessness, where a single dose of it can be taken late in the evening.
10. Do not administer *Lachesis* in frequent doses as it may lead the patient to the verge of incurable insanity.
11. Do not change the remedies too often. Allow them to work at least overnight in a majority of cases.
12. As far as possible, avoid eating and drinking for about half-an-hour before and after taking a homoeopathic medicine.

# 9 | COMMON AILMENTS AND THEIR HOMOEOPATHIC REMEDIES

## 1. ABDOMINAL PAIN

- When the food lies like a stone in the stomach and the patient feels better from rest. **Bry.** (11)
- When the abdomen is bloated, even after a light meal, with much flatulence and the patient is better by passing loud, noisy gas per anus. **Lyco.** (28)
- In case of gas and colic after eating, or after taking alcoholic beverages. **Nux-v.** (31)
- When the pains are violent and are relieved by bending double, heat and hard pressure. **Colo.** (17) *in alternation with* **Mag-p.** (29)
- When there are cutting pains in abdomen with beads of cold perspiration on forehead. **Verat.** (40)
- In case of cramping pains in abdomen. **Cupr.** (18)
- When the pains are intolerable. **Cham.** (15)

## 2. ABSCESS

- For unhealthy skin, when the matter has begun to form and the affected part is very sensitive to touch. **Hep.** (23)

- In case of abscess of the mouth, gum, and neck glands. **Merc.** (30)
- In inflammation with much soreness and blueness of the part. **Arn.** (7)
- During the inflammatory period, when there is throbbing pain and bright red swelling. **Bell.** (9) *in alternation with* **Merc.** (30)
- When the abscess has a shiny swollen appearance, with stinging and burning. **Apis** (6)
- When the part looks blue or purplish with hammering pain. **Lach.** (26)
- When the abscess has healed, to prevent recurrence. **Calc-p.** (12)

**Note :** Foment the abscess with hot water or dry heat. After the matter has been discharged, clean the wound with *Calendula lotion* (one teaspoonful of *Calendula* ϕ to two spoonfuls of water), dry it up and apply a bandage.

## 3. ACIDITY

- In case of severe burning in the food pipe after the intake of only a little food and when the condition becomes worse from cold food and cold drinks. **Lyco.** (28)
- For burning in chest and eructations. **Carb-v.** (14)
- For burning, tasteless eructations which are relieved by drinking hot water; flatulence with distension of the stomach, belching of gas and fullness in the stomach. **Mag-p.** (29)
- In case of infants with greenish diarrhoea and great restlessness. **Cham.** (15)

## 4. AMENORRHOEA

*(Menses absent, delayed, retarded, scanty, suppressed)*

- When the menses are suppressed by a chill or fright or sudden emotions.   **Acon.** (1)

- When the menses are irregular, suppressed, delayed and variable, from cold or getting the feet wet, or in damp, especially in the blouses with mild, yielding and weepy disposition.   **Puls.** (34)

- When the menses are suppressed by a chill or fright, or if there is nose-bleed in place of menses.   **Bry.** (11)

- In the full-blooded females, when the menses are suddenly suppressed, with colicky, throbbing pains in the lower abdomen; exhaustion and loss of appetite.   **Bell.** (9)

- When the menses are suppressed immediately after their onset and are often associated with shivering, nausea, vomiting, diarrhoea and profuse perspiration on face.   **Verat.** (40)

- In case of irregular periods, accompanying burning heat in the palms and soles. Pain in abdomen and loins, vertigo, throbbing head, and constipation; usually in obstinate cases.   **Sulph.** (39)

## 5. ANGINA PECTORIS *(Chest Pain)*

- In case of sudden severe pain about heart with throbbing and great sense of suffocation, anxiety and fear of death.   **Acon.** (1)

- When the patient feels a spasmodic choking and suffocative pain in the region of the heart.   **Arn.** (7) *in alternation with* **Mag.-p.** (29)

- When the pain is intolerable and compel the patient to walk on the floor. **Cham.** (15)
- In case of throbbing, stabbing pains about the heart with red face, especially when the pain is worse from the least jar. **Bell.** (9) *in alternation with* **Mag-p.** (29)
- When there is heaviness in the region of the heart, and violent, throbbing headache. **Glon.** (22)
- When the attacks are due to indigestion and are attended with, or followed by, gas and are worse on rising in the morning. **Nux-v.** (31)
- If the pains are accompanied with violent and visible palpitation of the heart. **Spig.** (37)

**Note :** As soon as an anginal attack is noticed, call in a doctor, and by the time he reaches, give one of the aforementioned medicines according to the symptoms.

## 6. ANXIETY

- For sudden panicky attacks with fear of death. **Acon.** (1)
- For awful anxiety, when the patient is excessively chilly and becomes so restless and prostrated that he can neither sit nor lie down, or stand at one place. **Ars.** (8)
- When the anxiety is associated with catarrh and cough. **Ipec.** (25)
- If accompanied with profuse sweat and empty, gone feeling in the stomach. **Sulph.** (40)
- If lacks self-confidence and needs reassurance. **Phos.** (32)
- In shy, anxious, emotional subjects, who suffer from intolerable heat and easily weep and symptoms are very changeable. **Puls.** (34)

## 7. APHTHAE, STOMATITIS *(small white ulcers and inflammation of mouth)*, SORE MOUTH

- When the tongue is dry, red, hot and acutely painful; with salivation and ulceration, diarrhoea and offensive breath.  **Merc. (30)**

- For dark-coloured eruptions, offensive odour from mouth, exhausting sickness and great debility.  **Ars. (8)** *to be followed by* **Carb-v. (14)**

- In case of canker sores, especially in children.  **Bor. (10)**

- When the tongue is red, granular and extremely painful.  **Bell. (9)**

- To prevent a relapse when the eruptions have nearly subsided or there is sour-smelling odour from the mouth.  **Sulph. (39)**

## 8. APPENDICULAR PAIN

- When the pain is of cutting character in the lower right abdominal region, worse on waking.  **Lach. (26)**

- When the pain is stinging or burning, and might have occurred after vaccination.  **Apis (6)**

- When there is burning pain, restlessness, thirst for sips of water, chill and exhaustion.  **Ars. (8)**

- When the patient lies motionless and the least movement or jar aggravates the pain.  **Bry. (11)**

- When the patient is restless, worse during rest and better from continued motion and warmth.  **Rhus-t. (35)**

## 9. APPETITE

- If there is ravenous hunger which varies to complete loss of appetite. **Ferr-p.** (20)

- If there is excessive hunger even at night, but which is quickly satisfied. **Lyco.** (28)

- When there is loss of appetite due to sedentary habits, study and swot, over-indulgence in spirituous liquors, or if there is complete aversion to food, but the patient is hungry in the evening and cannot sleep on this account. **Nux-v.** (31)

- If there is complete loss of appetite from partaking of rich food, pastry, pork, etc., or it is attended with loss of taste. **Puls.** (34)

## 10. ARTHRITIS *(Pain in joints)*

- When the large single joints of hands or small multiple joints of hands or feet are involved and the pain and stiffness are worse on sitting and during rest and in the morning on rising and better for heat and continued movements. **Rhus-t.** (35)

- When the joints are acutely painful and swollen and are worse from least movement or jar and better for rest and cold applications. **Bry.** (11)

- When heat is intolerable and the patient is thirstless, especially in those who are of mild, gentle and yielding nature. **Puls.** (34)

- When relief is noticed in mild, warm damp weather. **Ruta** (36)

## 11. ASTHMA

- In case of suffocative attacks and short anxious breathing, worse on lying down, with great distress, pale face, burning heat in chest, accompanied with great weakness, cold perspiration and prostration. **Ars.** (8)

- When there is frequent cough, with pain and soreness in the chest, or pain under the ribs. **Bry.** (11)

- If there is great tightness about the chest, with anxiety, or rattling in the chest from an accumulation of mucus, or in nightly attacks of suffocation, cold sweat, restlessness and nausea. **Ipec.** (25)

- When worse after a meal, or if there is a short cough with difficult discharge of phlegm and oppression in the lower part of the chest, and the clothes feel tight. **Nux-v.** (31)

- In individuals with excess of blood, with anxiety and difficult breathing, gored the exciting cause has been atmospheric, as fog, cold, dry air or chill. **Acon.** (1)

- In case of noisy, wheezy breathing, oppression, cough, if the patient is anxious and needs a lot of reassurance and attention. **Phos.** (32)

- For chronic cases, with a recurrence of cough; foul, thick mucoid, and unsatisfactory response to well-indicated remedies. **Sulph.** (39)

## 12. BACKACHE : See LUMBAGO.

## 13. BAD BREATH *(Halitosis)*

- When with a metallic taste in the mouth

and much sweating of the body, especially for one who can tolerate excess of neither heat nor cold. **Merc.** (30)

- When due to digestive upsets or in alcoholics, worse after a meal or in the morning. **Nux-v.** (31)
- When due to decaying teeth or infected gums, with flatulence, weakness and poor circulation of blood. **Carb-v.** (14)
- When associated with indigestion and marked changeability in the patient and the ailments. **Puls.** (34)
- When the tongue is coated white or yellow, with palpitation of heart. **Spig.** (37)
- In longstanding cases. **Sulph.** (39)

## 14. BED-WETTING

- When the urine is loaded with uric acid. **Lyco.** (28)
- In case of nervous, hysterical children. **Gels.** (21)
- When the bed wetting occurs in the early night hours. **Bell.** (9)
- When the urine has a coffee smell and there is often involuntary escape while coughing and weakness of Sphincter muscle. **Ferr-p.** (21)
- For the over-conscious child, who is thin, chilly and excessively anxious, i.e., an obsessional personality. **Ars.** (8)

## 15. BILIOUS ATTACKS *(diseases from excessive secretion of bile)*

- When accompanied by headache, dryness of mouth and lips, distended stomach,

- vomiting after drinking or eating, and the food lying heavily in the stomach like a stone, with much thirst.    *Bry.* (11)
- If brought on by anger, grief, chagrin and the nausea is intensified even by thought, sight or smell of food.    *Cocc.* (16)
- When due to over-eating or taking too much alcoholic beverages, or coffee, resulting in sour taste and nausea after eating and in the morning, with much retching and gagging as well as great giddiness, with constipation and crampy headache.    *Nux-v.* (31)
- In case of severe and persisting nausea and vomiting, abundant flow of watery saliva, shivering and shuddering, and headache as if the head, bruised.    *Ipec.* (25)
- When the tongue is yellow and the complexion is dirty.    *Merc.* (30)
- For headache with nausea and soreness of the scalp.    *Ferr-p.* (20)
- When the bowels are relaxed and there is chilliness, and the attack has been caused by rich or fat food, or pork.    *Puls.* (34)

## 16. BILIOUS COLIC

- If the colic is very severe, with spasmodic, crampy feeling in the bowels, or if they are distended and feel very tender.    *Cham.* (15)
- If there are shooting or violent pinching pains, especially in the centre of the abdomen, with nausea.    *Merc.* (30)
- In case of violent cramp-like pains, constipation, or pains and weariness in the thighs.    *Nux-v.* (31)

- If there are spasmodic or cutting pains or looseness of bowels, or shivering. ***Puls.*** (34)

## 17. BILIOUS DIARRHOEA

- If very violent, with great loss of strength and thirst for frequent sips of water. ***Ars.*** (8)
- If the evacuation is like stirred-up eggs and there is much pain. ***Cham.*** (15)
- In ordinary cases of bilious diarrhoea, with great tenesmus before, during and after stools. ***Merc.*** (30)
- If there are watery, green or bilious, slimy stools arising from indigestion or stomach upset. ***Puls.*** (34)

## 18. BILIOUS HEADACHE

- In case of great nausea and vomiting and bruised feeling in head. ***Ipec.*** (25)
- When the pains seem as though a nail were driven into the head; or when there is giddiness, confusion and faintness; or if the headache is worse in the open air. ***Nux-v.*** (31)
- If there are one-sided (semi-lateral) pains, which are relieved by compression, or by being in the open air. ***Puls.*** (34)
- In case of violent headache, with vomiting and pale face, or with throbbing pains. ***Verat.*** (40)

## 19. BITES & STINGS

- For stings of bees, wasps, hornets, with burning, stinging pains and rapid, rosy, watery swelling. ***Apis*** (6)

- If the part is very red, toughened and burning. **Canth.** (13)
- In case of bites by rats, scorpions, mosquitoes, with coldness, swelling and numbness of the parts, with relief from cold applications (and also to prevent bad effects of bites, swellings, etc.). **Led.** (27)
- In case of rat-bites when the pain shoots from below upwards. **Hyper.** (24)
- If the tongue is stung by a bee, or when the eye is stung. **Acon.** (1)
  *in alternation with*
  **Arn.** (7)
- In the event of bite by a mad dog. **Bell.** (9)
  *in alternation with*
  **Hyper.** (24)
- If bitten by a snake. **Lach.** (26)

## 20. BLACK-EYE

- To lessen the bruising and swelling. **Arn.** (7)
  *in alternation with*
  **Led.** (27)
- When there is severe bruising of the surrounding muscles and face. **Ruta** (36)

## 21. BLADDER, PAINFUL

- When accompanied by burning pains, with frequent desire to urinate; difficult urination. **Canth.** (13)
- When the pains are relieved by hard pressure or bending double. **Colo.** (17)

## 22. BLEEDING

See HAEMORRHAGES.

## 23. BLEEDING FROM CUTS

- In case of arterial bleeding or collapse. **Arn.** (7)

Note : Apply *Calendula* locally. If the bleeding is severe the part may be tied up tightly and the patient rushed to the nearest hospital to have surgical aid.

## 23. BLEEDING FROM NOSE : See *EPISTAXIS*

## 24. BLEEDING FROM URINARY ORGANS

- Discharge of pure blood in drops, or copiously blended with urine, especially when associated with difficulty in passing water, scalding urine and spasmodic pains. **Canth.** (13)
- In case of bleeding from external violence, strains, fall or severe efforts. **Arn.** (7) *in alternation with* **Acon.** (1)

## 25. BLEPHARITIS: See *Eyelids, Inflammation of*

## 26. BLOOD POISONING

- Blood poisoning occurring from any cause. **Lach.** (26)

## 27. BLOOD PRESSURE, HIGH *(Hypertension)*

- When attended with bursting headache, sleeplessness and tossing-about; pulse full and bounding; vertigo, worse on rising. **Acon.** (1)
- When attended with suppressed or scanty or high-coloured urine, loaded with casts, thirstlessness. **Apis** (6)
- For plethoric full-blooded people who have a tendency to haemorrhage; vertigo. **Arn.** (7)

- When attended with great anguish and restlessness, wheezing respiration, palpitation, great thirst for sips of water. **Ars.** (8)
- If associated with hot, red and flushed face, glaring eyes, headache, throbbing carotids, excited mental states and vertigo, with tendency to fall to the left side or backward. **Bell.** (9)
- When the head feels enormously large, with surging of blood to head and heart; confusion and dizziness. **Glon.** (22)

## 28. BLOOD PRESSURE, LOW *(Hypotension)*

- When blood seems to stagnate in the capillaries and the patient is sluggish, fat and lazy, debilitated, and craves fresh air. **Carb-v.** (14)
- If associated with general prostration, dizziness, dullness and drowsiness and trembling; vertigo, spreading from the occiput (back of head) over the whole head. **Gels.** (21)

## 29. BLOOD SPITTING *or* VOMITING

- When accompanied by flushed face, palpitation, anguish, shivering, quick pulse, great restlessness and fear of death. **Acon.** (1)
- When from a fall, a blow or severe exertion. **Arn.** (7)
 *in alternation with*
 **Acon.** (1)
- When associated with paleness of the face and frequent inclination to vomit, or when accompanied with short cough and expectoration streaked with blood. **Ipec.** (25)
- In case of difficulty in breathing, extreme

palpitation of the heart, burning heat and thirst, small and quick pulse. **Ars.** *(8)*

## 30. BLUSHING *(Red Glow of Skin)*

- For easy blushing with beads of sweat, just above the upper lip, in thin, outgoing but nervous and oversensitive adolescents. **Phos.** *(32)*
- For blushing of emotional origin in shy adolescents, who easily burst into tears and need sympathy. **Puls.** *(34)*
- For pallor with quick flushing in new or tense situations. **Ferr-p.** *(20)*

## 31. BODY ODOUR

- In case of profuse sour, sticky sweat day and night, with skin very sensitive to touch. **Hep.** *(23)*
- When with profuse offensive perspiration which stains the clothes yellow. **Merc.** *(30)*
- In case of profuse offensive sweat following an exercise or emotion. **Nux-v.** *(31)*

## 32. BOILS

- If the boil is burning hot and painful with a red, shining, inflamed base and much throbbing pain. **Bell.** *(9)* *in alternation with* **Merc.** *(30)*
- In case of summer boils or when the boils appear in crops. **Arn.** *(7)*
- To mature the boil when suppuration has commenced; very useful to clear the system. **Hep.** *(23)*

- When the boils threaten to become putrid and suppurate. **Merc.** (30)
- To prevent a recurrence of boils. **Sulph.** (39)
  *to be followed by*
  **Calc-p.** (12)

Note: Be careful with the diet. Avoid salt, meat, acids and spirits. Foment the boils with hot water.

## 33. BONES

- For all kinds of fractures, or when the children's bones do not grow firm, or when the fractures are slow to heal and the refuse to unite. **Calc-p.** (12)
- In case of injuries to ribs and periosteum (bone covering) of the bones. **Ruta** (36)

## 34. BREAST ABSCESS

- In the early stages, when there is severe pain, restlessness, often with high fever. **Acon.** (1)
- When the breast is hot and inflamed, usually with a raised body temperature. **Bell.** (9)
- When the breast is hard and tense. **Bry.** (11)

## 35. BREAST FEEDING

- When due to excess of milk in the breasts, they are tense, swollen and painful with weeping disposition and intolerance of heat. **Puls.** (34)
- When the breasts overflow in between the feeds. **Bor.** (10)
- When the milk decreases in the breasts due to fear or shock. **Acon.** (1)
- When the milk decreases due to anger. **Cham.** (15)

## 36. BREASTS, INFLAMMATION OF: See MASTITIS.

## 37. BREASTS, PAINFUL

- When the breasts are painful, heavy and red with a sensation of heat. **Bell.** (9)
- If the breasts are heavy and painful but without redness and inflammation. **Bry.** (11)
- When the breasts are swollen and painful whether in pregnancy or after it. **Puls.** (34)
- When the breasts are so painful as likely to ulcerate at every menstrual period. **Merc.** (30)

## 38. BREATH, OFFENSIVE

See BAD BREATH.

## 39. BREATHING DIFFICULTY

- When the patient is compelled to sit up or bend forward to get relief. **Ars.** (8)
- If associated with a dry throat and wheezing respiration and the patient feels better lying on the right side. **Bry.** (11)
- In children and old persons with respiratory troubles. **Ant-t.** (5)

## 40. BRONCHITIS

- For rattling of mucus in the bronchial tubes, nausea, etc. **Ipec.** (25)
- For inflammatory stage, with fever, short dry cough and constant irritation in the throat, chest and trachea, great restless-

ness, anxiety and fever, usually due to exposure to cold winds. **Acon.** (1)

- In children and old persons, with wheezy, difficult breathing and rattling of mucus in the chest, which cannot be raised; marked exhaustion. **Ant-t.** (5)

- When there are stitches in the right side of chest, or pain in the head on coughing, with wheezing and heavy respiration, or if there is a painful, violent dry cough, with headache and pain in the chest walls, better by supporting the painful part with hands. **Bry.** (11)

- When the mucus-rattle is prominent, the skin is hot and dry, and efforts to expectorate are ineffectual. **Hep.** (23)

- If there are pains in the chest or throat, great hoarseness, or a dry cough from tickling in the throat, tight breath with wheezing, worse from talking and fresh air. **Phos.** (32)

- If there is much hoarseness, with hollow, barking, dry cough, wheezing and sawing breath, or burning in chest. **Spong.** (38)

- In case of high temperature, dry cough, pulsating headache, a flushed face with a dry, hot skin, and when the cough is worse at night and by lying down. **Bell.** (9)

## 41. BRUISES

- In case of bruises of soft parts, caused due to injuries from a blow or fall. **Arn.** (7)

- When the bruised parts are rich in nerves, such as finger-tips, nail-beds, palms, soles, tail-bone (coccyx), etc. **Hyper.** (24)

- If there is more of sprain than bruises, and if it is more external and painful to touch, with great restlessness. **Rhus-t.** (35)
- For bruises about the eyes from blows with fist, stick, stone, flying cork, etc. **Led.** (27) *in alternation with* **Arn.** (7)
- If the periosteum (bone covering) is involved. **Ruta.** (36)

Note : If the skin is broken, wash the part with *Calendula* lotion.

## 42. BURNS & SCALDS

- To prevent nervous shock, and fear of death. **Acon.** (1)
- To prevent shock and burning pains. **Arn.** (7) *in alternation with* **Bell.** (9)
- If the burning pains persist, or when there is formation of vesicle blisters, the skin is red and peeling. **Canth.** (13) *in alternation with* **Bell.** (9)
- In case of intolerable pains, with a tendency to convulsions. **Cham.** (15)
- When parts are actually painful, fiery red and burning, with high temperature. **Bell.** (9) *in alternation with* **Ferr-p.** (20)
- When suppuration takes place. **Hep.** (23)
- When vesicles turn black, showing a tendency to gangrene. **Ars.** (8)
- In case of mild burns and scalds, the skin being bright or scarlet red and swollen. **Sulph.** (39) (usually follows *Cantharis*).

Note : Apply *Cantharis* ϕ directly to a burn before blisters are formed. In case of severe burns, rush the patient immediately to hospital. Meanwhile, give *Acon.* (1) and *Arn.* (7) internally in alternation to prevent shock and fear of death.

## 43. CAR SICKNESS: See MOTION SICKNESS

## 44. CATARRHAL FEVER : See FEVERS.

## 45. CATARRH: See COLDS.

## 46. CHANGE OF LIFE *(Menopause)*

- For fair, blue-eyed women, with mild, yielding disposition. **Puls.** (34)
- For flushes of heat. **Lach.** (26)

## 47. CHICKEN POX

- At the onset of the symptoms, when there is great restlessness of body and mind. **Rhus-t.** (35)
- For fever and congestion. **Ferr-p.** (20)
- If the brain is affected, or when there is much heat or pain in the brain, flushing, sore throat and fever. **Bell.** (9)
- If there is much itching. **Merc.** (30)
- In case the child is mild, tearful and thirstless and the eruption is slow in its development, or there are gastric symptoms. **Puls.** (34)
- In fever, with symptoms of anxiety, fear, thirst, dry heat, rapid, hard and full pulse. **Acon.** (1)
- In case of excessive itching, burning and heat of the eruptions. **Apis** (6)
- When the eruption in slow to form, with cough and cold. **Ant-t.** (5)
- When the fever is slow to fall and the patient is weak, drowsy and dizzy. **Gels.** (21)

- To prevent relapse during the period of convalescence. **Calc-p.** (12)

## 48. CHILBLAINS

*(Painful swelling with redness of hands and feet during winter.)*

- When there is intolerable itching, swelling and stinging pain, worse from heat. **Apis** (6)
- In case of hard, shining skin, bruised pain and itching of the parts. **Arn.** (7)
- In case of inflammation, pulsative pains, fiery redness and swelling of the skin. **Bell.** (9)
- When the chilblains itch and burn, especially from warmth of bed. **Carb-v.** (14)
- When the burning pains are accompanied by ulceration, especially in emaciated children. **Ars.** (8)
- When caused by frosted feet and the affected part is bluish, with pricking-burning pain, and is worse from heat, in the evening and letting the limb hang down. **Puls.** (34)
- If there is much pain and inflammation. **Ferr-p.** (20)
- When the chilblains occur in persons having a defective circulation and nutritional deficiency. **Calc-p.** (12)
- For obstinate type of chilblains of blue-red colour, with itching, aggravated by warmth and cold bath. **Sulph.** (39)

**Note :** In case of broken skin, the part should be thoroughly cleaned with *Calendula* lotion and, later on, *Coconut oil* may be applied when dry.

## 49. CHILD-BIRTH

- In case of great fear and anxiety. **Acon.** (1)
- To abort bruised feeling after child-birth. **Arn.** (7)
- In case of malposition of the foetus. **Puls.** (34)
- If labour is unduly prolonged and the abdomen is strained. **Rhus-t.** (35)
- In case of frequent urging for stool or urination. **Nux-v.** (31)

## 50. CHOLERA

- When due to too free indulgence in fruits or ice; purging and vomiting frequently with intense burning pains or cramps in the stomach and bowels, with violent thirst for sips of water, great prostration and restlessness. **Ars.** (8)
- When the evacuations are profuse both upward and downward; the stools are watery, frothy, and the features are sunken, with profuse cold sweat on forehead, great thirst and cramps in hands and feet. **Verat.** (40)
- When there is complete collapse, with coldness of breath in the last stage, but the patient wants to be continually fanned. **Carb-v.** (14)
- When the cramps are more severe, especially in the arms and legs. **Cupr.** (18)
- When first symptoms of diarrhoea appear during an epidemic. **Sulph.** (39)

## 51. COLDS & CATARRHS *(discharges)*

- In case of sudden onset after exposure to dry, cold winds, with frequent dry sneezing, burning of the throat and mouth, fever, thirst, restlessness at night and buzzing in the ears, worse in stuffy atmosphere.    ***Acon.*** (1) *in alternation with* ***Ferr-p.*** (20)

- In case of paroxysms of sneezing, corroding watery discharge from the nostrils, making the nose and upper lip sore, raw and painful; rawness in the throat and chest, worse in a warm room, better in fresh open air.    ***All-c.*** (3)

- When there is copious thick yellow discharge from the nose, with frequent sneezing, foul breath and discharge of greenish-yellow mucus on coughing, often with enlarged and tender cervical glands, sweating with severe infection of throat and febrile symptoms.    ***Merc.*** (30)

- When the patient is chilly and catches cold with every change of weather with frequent sneezing and abundant thin, hot, excoriating, burning watery discharge from the eyes and nose, with lassitude and great prostration; nostrils very sore great prostration.    ***Ars.*** (8)

- In case of very violent onset after exposure, especially of head; nose swollen, sore, red and hot; throat raw, sore and hoarse; face red and hot.    ***Bell.*** (9)

- If there is watery discharge from the nose, especially in case of colds of infants.    ***Cham.*** (15)

- When with delayed onset, much sneezing, eyes red and watery discharge from the nose, dryness of mouth and lips; dry stuffy nose, harsh, hard, dry painful and shaking cough with stitch-like pain in the sides and chest, severe headache, worse from cold and motion; thirst for large quantities of cold water at long intervals; holds the chest and head when coughing.    ***Bry.*** (11)

**COLD & CATARRHS**      **COLD CATARRHS**

# COMMON AILMENTS AND THEIR REMEDIES

- In the early stages without very marked indications. ***Ferr-p.*** (20)

- In influenzal type of cold, in warm moist, or change of, weather, corroding watery discharge from the nose with sneezing, hot and dry throat, headache with heavy eyes and chills running up and down the spine with shivering; no thirst even during fever. ***Gels.*** (21)

- For colds which come on in dry, cold weather in its early stages; much sneezing, nose running the whole day and stuffed up at night, better outdoors; constipation, backache and irritability; the child cannot suck due to blocking of nostrils. ***Nux-v.*** (31)

- If there is violent catarrh, with great hoarseness, pain in the chest and cough. ***Phos.*** (32)

- For cold in damp weather or getting wet. ***Rhus-t.*** (35)

- When the discharge from the nose is bland or offensive, and tears are acrid. ***Euphr.*** (19)

- In case of variable symptoms, with thick, greenish-yellow discharge from the nose, or when there is complete loss of taste and smell, worse in the evening, in a warm room and at night, better in a cool room with windows open for fresh air. ***Puls.*** (34)

- In case of copious burning, excoriating, clear watery discharge from the nose, chilliness, craving for heat, great prostration, agitation, sneezing and watering eyes. ***Ars.*** (8)

- In case of chronic catarrh, with free discharge, burning heat in palms and soles. ***Sulph.*** (39)

- To build up the general health after colds. ***Calc-p.*** (12)

## 52. COLIC *(Enteralgia)*

- When there is much colic-like clutching, or sensation as if the bowels were grasped with nails and the pain is aggravated by pressure or jar and relief is obtained by bending or leaning forward. *Bell.* (9)

- When the pain is worse by least movement, jar and heat and better lying motionless on back, with knees drawn up. *Bry.* (11)

- In case of colic, especially from a chill, with intolerable twisting, pinching pain in stomach, tearing around navel, under short ribs; colic of teething children, with legs drawn up, red face and irritability; the pain is better by application of local heat and at night. *Cham.* (15)

- When the patient suffers from violent, cutting, tearing and griping pains in the stomach with flatulence (gas), tenesmus (straining of bowels) and diarrhoea; can't keep still and finds relief from hard pressure, bending double and passing wind. *Colo.* (17) *in alternation with* *Mag-p.* (29)

- If due to constipation, or from indigestion due to overeating; when the pains are cramping, pinching or spasmodic; or it is cutting pain in urinary bladder, better by sitting or lying down. *Nux-v.* (31)

- When there is a feeling of congestion in the abdomen, and the colic is very violent, cramp-like and sudden. *Acon.* (1)

- If the pain is in the upper part of the stomach with flatulence, which is not relieved by belching. *Carb-v.* (14)

- When hot applications relieve pain. *Mag-p.* (29)

- In case of severe colicky pain with blueness of skin and face, cold sweat on forehead,

- tenderness and distension (swelling) of the abdomen and symptoms of collapse; the pain is relieved by bowel motion. *Verat.* (40)
- If there are cramp-like spasmodic pains with nausea or faintness, wind, or pressive pains and spasms in the chest, or violent pains relieved by emission of wind. *Cocc.* (16)
- When the colic is oppressive and the pains are worse on sitting or lying down, or with disagreeable tension in the abdomen. *Puls.* (34)
- If there are shooting or violent contracting pains, especially around the navel, with much tenderness of the abdomen; colic due to worms. *Merc.* (30)
- When the pain is in the pit of stomach, associated with nausea, restlessness and often worse for the least movement. *Ipec.* (25)
- In case of colic radiating upwards and it is relieved by applying local heat. *Mag-p.* (29)

## 53. COLLAPSE & SHOCK

- To prevent a shock due to an accident, injury, burn, etc., with fear of death. *Acon.* (1) *in alternation with* *Arn.* (7)
- When there is great hunger for air, desire to be fanned, coldness of whole body, cold breath and mental torpor. *Carb-v.* (14)
- When the skin is marble-cold and there are beads of cold sweat on the forehead; the face is pale, blue and collapsed; the features are sunken, Hippocratic. *Verat.* (40)
- In case of great uneasiness, oppressed breathing, prostration, thirst and craving for warmth. *Ars.* (8)

## 54. CONJUNCTIVITIS *(ophthalmia)*

- For acute inflammation of eyes, especially after injuries or operation. **Acon.** (1)

- For pain, redness and swelling, throbbing in temples (sides of head), flushed cheeks, glistening eyes and intolerance of light. **Bell.** (9) *in alternation with* **Ferr-p.** (20)

- With inability to bear bright light. **Euphr.** (19)

- In patients of measles and gonorrhoea, accompanied with bland, yellowish discharge from the eyes, with itching; worse in the evening and better in open air. **Puls.** (34)

- If there is oedematous soft swelling of eyelids, with heat, stinging pain and hot tears. **Apis** (6)

- When the lids are convulsively closed and if forced open, hot scalding tears gush out from the eyes. **Rhus-t.** (35)

- In chronic scrofulous ophthalmia. **Hep.** (23) *in alternation with* **Merc.** (30)

- To prevent frequent relapses. **Calc-p.** (12) *& occasional doses of* **Sulph.** (39)

## 55. CONSTIPATION

- When the stools are large-sized, hard, dry, as if burnt, passed with great difficulty; chilliness, irritability and headache, worse movement. **Bry.** (11)

- When with frequent ineffectual urging for stool, nausea and sickness, especially in persons of lazy habits and those taking laxatives regularly to move the bowels. **Nux-v.** (31)

## COMMON AILMENTS AND THEIR REMEDIES

- When the stool is evacuated with great straining. **Ruta. (36)**

- In case of tightness and itching of the anus, rumbling and flatulence in the abdomen, gush of acid fluids into the mouth from stomach with heartburn (burning of gullet), loaded urine, etc. **Lyco. (28)**

- If there is bitter or metallic taste in the mouth, but no loss of appetite, or when the evacuations are lumpy, or passed in one solid ball, dark-coloured, dry or covered with mucus. **Merc. (30)**

- For habitual costiveness. **Sulph. (39)** *in the morning and* **Nux-v. (31)** *at bed time*

### 56. CONTUSED WOUNDS: See BRUISES.

### 57. CONVALESCENCE

- To restore the quality of blood, to aid assimilation and to tone up the general system. **Calc-p. (12)** *may be alternated with* **Ferr-p. (20)**

### 58. CONVULSIONS: See FITS.

### 59. COUGH

- In the beginning of a cold, accompanied with constant hard, dry, cramp-like cough with flushed face, headache, thirst, anxiety, restlessness, constipation and a feeling of suffocation, especially after exposure to dry, cold winds; worse at night and better for cold. **Acon. (1)**

- When accompanied by wheezing respiration, much frothy phlegm, restlessness and anxiety, weakness and great prostration, worse after midnight; acid, bitter, frothy or salty expectoration. **Ars. (8)**

- When the cough is spasmodic, shaking, suffocating, hard, dry and painful, and seems to burst open the head or chest, when the patient has to hold the head or chest during coughing, with great dryness of throat or larynx or when the cough ends in sneezing or a whoop, or when the patient desires large quantities of cold water. **Bry. (11)** *in alternation with* **Mag-p. (29)**

- For violent spells of hard and dry cough, which bring up a lump of phlegm or are followed by retching and gagging, with very red face. **Carb-v. (14)**

- In case of sudden, spasmodic, incessant, continuous, suffocative, moist cough, with rattling respiration, often associated with wheezing and a sensation of weight in the chest; intense nausea and vomiting. The child may turn blue and go stiff. **Ipec. (25)**

- For short, dry, shaking and paroxysmal cough, dryness of larynx, headache, flushed face, worse at night. **Bell. (9)**

- In case of dry, teasing or spasmodic cough, with gagging and retching; feverish and desperately chilly; bruised feeling in the stomach on coughing; violent headache during coughing. **Nux-v. (31)**

- For dry, teasing cough, with tickling deep down in air tubes, worse at night, uncovering; restlessness, must keep moving. **Rhus-t. (35)**

- When there is bleeding from the nose or spitting of blood with each fit of coughing (especially in whooping cough). The child cries before the cough begins. **Arn. (7)**

- In case of great exhaustion, cold perspiration, vomiting and involuntary escape of urine during cough. ***Verat.*** (40)
- For hard, dry, hollow, convulsive or spasmodic cough, with great dryness, of respiratory tract; face red during cough, frontal headache, worse in the evening and sensation of tickling in the throat. ***Bell.*** (9) *in alternation with* ***Ferr-p.*** (20)
- When the cough is worse on lying down, after eating and in the evening; with disgusting, frothy mucus, thick or profuse expectoration. ***Puls*** (34)
- When the cough is irritating, worse in the evening, before midnight (preventing sleep) and in the morning, with hoarseness, raw feeling in the chest, dry cough excited by tickling in throat, with rust-coloured, bloody and pus-like mucus raised; great soreness and pain in the chest on coughing. ***Phos.*** (32)
- When the cough is due to infection (most likely bronchitis), moist and loose, or when with wheezing, air hunger and weakness, or when the cough is accompanied by thick, yellowish green discharge. ***Hep.*** (23)
- For shaking cough accompanied by acrid or watery phlegm, with sore throat and hoarseness. ***Merc.*** (30)
- For a dry irritating cough, often provoked by a fit of anger; or cough in children during dentition, with irritability, wheezing breath, fretfulness and restlessness. ***Cham.*** (15)
- When there is a dry, barking, whistling cough, with tickling, hoarseness and loss of voice, better after eating and drinking. ***Spong.*** (38)
- When the cough is only during daytime. ***Euphr.*** (19)
- In case of obstinate cough with dirty-

looking, thick, greenish-yellow or copious mucus expelled; moist and rattling respiration. *Sulph.* (39)

See also **WHOOPING COUGH.**

## 60. CRAMPS

- When the fingers, legs and toes are especially involved. *Cupr.* (18)
- For paroxysmal cramps, spasms, neuralgia (nerve-pains), twitchings, etc. *Mag-p.* (29)
- In case of sensation as if parts were asleep, with a feeling of numbness and coldness. *Calc-p.* (12)
- In very acute and severe cases of cramps in legs and thighs, particularly at night. *Cham.* (15)
- If the cramps are very violent in calf muscles and are accompanied with coldness of feet, better by local massage and worse by walking about. *Verat.* (40)
- When the cramps and spasms are generally worse from 2 to 3 a.m., and are associated with headache, loss of appetite, nausea, indigestion and constipation (generally with frequent urging for stool) and irritability. *Nux-v.* (31)
- When there are burning pains of arms and legs, writer's cramps, better on moving the affected parts; irritability. *Gels.* (21)

## 61. CROUP *(disease of larynx with laborious breathing)*

- In case of hoarse, hollow cough, with wheezing, rattling of mucus in the chest and suffocative feeling on lying down. *Hep.* (23)

## COMMON AILMENTS AND THEIR REMEDIES

- During the inflammatory period, when there is fever, with short dry cough, and hurried breathing. **Acon. (1)**
- When there is hoarse, hollow, barking and crowing cough, or slow loud wheezing and sawing respiration, or fits of choking. **Spong. (38)**

## 62. CRYING OF INFANTS

- If the skin is hot and dry, and the child is restless and sleepless. **Acon. (1)**
- When the head is hot and eyes congested; child suddenly starts in sleep and cries for no perceptible reason. **Bell. (9)**
- When the child cries due to troublesome teething or with stomach upset, and there is headache, earache, acidity, etc. **Cham. (15)**
- When due to colic from indigestion, with frequent urging for stool. **Nux-v. (31)**
- When due to hunger on account of vomiting of curdled milk. **Aeth-Co. (2)**
- When the baby cries all the day but sleeps the whole night. **Lyco. (28)**

## 63. CUTS: See WOUNDS.

## 64. DANDRUFF

- When there is a lot of flaking and scaling and very dry skin. **Lyco. (28)**
- In case of dry, flaking skin in chilly and exhausted subjects. **Ars. (8)**
- If there is associated acne, flaking and itching. **Sulph. (39)**

## 65. DENTIST

- Before and after visiting, or getting the teeth examined by a dental surgeon, or before tooth extraction. **Arn.** (7)

## 66. DENTITION (teething)

- In case of much diarrhoea, with feverishness, redness, pain, swelling of gums, restlessness and intense thirst. **Acon.** (1)
- In case of convulsions during dentition with congestion of head, redness of face and eyes, and irritability. **Bell.** (9)
- When the child is peevish, cross, obstinate or ugly; shrieks and angrily cries when touched or looked at, or when there are dry cough, short breathing, fretfulness, one cheek pale and the other flushed, loose green or frothy stools and irritability of the child. **Cham.** (15)
- In case the child is constipated and suffers from painful and frequent urging for stool. **Nux-v.** (31)
- When teeth sprout slowly and decay rapidly, and sutures in skull edges are wide open. **Calc-p.** (12)
- In case of sufferings in head, sleeplessness, crying out and tossing about, dullness, drowsiness and dizziness. **Gels.** (21)
- If colic is present and the child feels better by pressing the abdomen. **Colo.** (17)

## 67. DIARRHOEA

- When brought on by exposure to cold, dry winds or as a result of fright. **Acon.** (1)

- When accompanied by colicky pains, involuntary profuse watery stools after taking least food or drinks, sense of insecurity at anus and rumbling of gas in the abdomen. **Aloes** (4)
- For diarrhoea as a complication of shock or injury. **Arn.** (7)
- In very severe cases of diarrhoea, with violent colicky pains, or great prostration (loss of strength), resulting from eating fruit and vegetables, alcoholic beverages, ice-creams or taking icy cold drinks when hot, or taking tainted food; stools burning, watery, with much mucus, and often green or pale in colour, and nearly always associated with vomiting, collapse and chill. **Ars.** (8)
- If resulting from the heat of summer, eating sour fruits, or drinking cold water when overheated; early morning diarrhoea, driving the patient out of bed; dry parched lips. **Bry.** (11)
- For dentitional diarrhoea in infants, restlessness, crossness, fretfulness and severe colicky pain in the abdomen, grass-green stools which contain particles of undigested food, mucus and blood and smell like rotten eggs. **Cham.** (15)
- In case of brown, watery, or faecal diarrhoea, attended with severe colicky pains, which are somewhat relieved by hard pressure and bending double. **Colo.** (17)
- When with painless evacuations, or debility and emaciation. **Phos.** (32)
- If occurring in the heat of summer or in the autumn, with fermented, green or yellow stools which are of a very offensive smelling. **Ipec.** (25)

**DIARRHOEA**      **DIARRHOEA**

- If the stools are of green colour and mixed with mucus and there is much painful straining. *Merc.* (30)

- When the stools are changeable and variable, and are worse in the evening, following rich, starchy, fatty food, pastries, etc. *Puls.* (34)

- For painful diarrhoea of old people, with frequent involuntary cadaverous smelling stools, accompanied by great prostration. *Carb-v.* (14)

- For early morning watery diarrhoea, driving the patient out of bed, with sensation as if the bowels were too weak to retain their contents. *Sulph.* (39)

- If due to over-indulgence in food, with frequent urging for stool and pain in the abdomen before passing stools. *Nux-v.* (31)

- If accompanied by vomiting, great debility, severe cutting pains in the abdomen, profuse cold sweat on forehead, with great thirst for icy-cold water and desire to keep the windows wide open. *Verat.* (40)

- For diarrhoea caused by fright and other emotional upsets, exciting news and anticipation of any unusual ordeals, or to meet an engagement. *Gels.* (21)

- When with coldness, collapse and cramps in the abdomen and the calves of legs. *Cupr.* (18)

- In case of undigested stools, and to tone up general health. *Ferr-p.* (20) in alternation with *Calc-p.* (12)

## 68. DIPHTHERIA

- When the throat is intensely swollen. *Apis* (6)

# COMMON AILMENTS AND THEIR REMEDIES

- When beginning on the left side of throat and extending to the right side. **Lach. (26)**
- When beginning on the right side and extending to the left side. **Lyco. (28)**

## 69. DIZZINESS: See VERTIGO.

## 70. DYSENTERY

- In case of very sudden and acute onset in hot weather or hot climate, with great restlessness and fear of death. **Acon. (1)**
- When attended with shreddy, bloodstained stools, with great straining, burning and tenesmus in the abdomen and painful urination. **Canth. (13)**
- When attended with severe griping, colicky pains which are relieved by hard pressure and bending double. **Colo. (17)**
- For autumnal dysentery, when accompanied by severe straining, colic, nausea and vomiting, constant call for stool, but cannot get off the pain; very slimy stools in the beginning, followed by bloody stools. **Ipec. (25)**
- When the stools are small, bloody, mixed with mucus, accompanied by severe cutting pains in the abdomen and frequent urging for stools, worse in morning on rising. **Nux-v. (31)**
- If there is violent straining, with bloody evacuations, mixed with mucus, clammy perspiration and shivering; pain after stool. **Merc. (30)**
- In case of bloody stools, with burning thirst and severe cutting pains in the abdomen

and frequent urging to defecate, coldness of extremities, cold breath, putrid and offensive involuntary urine. **Ars.** (8)

## 71. DYSMENORRHOEA: *See MENSES, PAINFUL.*

## 72. EARACHE *(otalgia)*

- For sudden, acute earache after a chill or exposure to cold or cold winds, with red, hot face, fever, violent pain, relieved by local heat. **Acon.** (1)
- For nerve pains (neuralgia), accompanied by coryza, or in post-discharge stages. **All-c.** (3)
- In case of digging, beating, throbbing, tearing, shooting pains, often in right ear, sometimes extending to throat with headache and is worse by least jar, or noise, and better by heat and lying flat on back; thirstlessness; the child cries out in sleep. **Bell.** (9)
- When the pain arises from a chill and is very severe, pricking and of stabbing character, almost intolerable, and gets worse from local heat and better by carrying, especially in irritable, cross and fretful children. **Cham.** (15)
- When there is much inflammation with darting, tearing and variable pain and sensation, as if something would pass through the ear. **Puls.** (34)
- When the pain is of a neuralgic character, especially if it is periodical. **Gels.** (21)
- When there is much chilliness, with throbbing shooting pains extending to teeth, throbbing worse in warm bed; enlarged glands. **Merc.** (30)

COMMON AILMENTS AND THEIR REMEDIES 55

- For stitching pains, sore-throat; chilly, peevish and irritable subjects; worse from the least draught; the pain generally starts in the left ear and then moves to the right ear. *Hep.* (23)
- When the bones around the ear ache and there is some swelling. *Calc-p.* (12)

Note : Instil a drop of *Plantago major* φ in the affected ear to have instant relief.

## 73. EARS, DISCHARGE FROM: See *OTORRHOEA*.

## 74. EARS, HUMMING IN THE *(Tinnitus)*

- In case of humming noises, irritation and high-pitched ringing in the ears, generally arising from congestion of blood to the head, with great agitation of mind and body. *Bell.* (9)
- If from indigestion, or if worse in the morning. *Nux-v.* (31)
- If from indigestion or chill, or if worse in the evening. *Puls.* (34)
- For roaring, singing sounds in the ears, better from shaking the ears with finger. *Lach.* (26)
- When there is heat and oversensitiveness to noise, especially in anaemic subjects. *Ferr-p.* (20)
- In obstinate cases when there are humming and gurgling noises in the ears. *Sulph.* (39)

## 75. EARS, INFLAMMATION OF *(Otitis)*

- In case of acute pain, with high fever and great restlessness; externally the ear is red, hot, swollen and painful. *Acon.* (1)

EARACHE              EARS, INFLAMMATION

- When there is great irritability, and beating, throbbing pain deep in the ear, which extends to the throat; fever with extreme sensibility to noise; pain causes delirium; the child cries out in sleep. *Bell.* (9)

- If there is severe pain, high temperature, swelling of the glands, or soreness and sensation of icy cold water in the ear, and discharge of pus; the child is restless, crying, often sweating and, maybe, delirious. *Merc.* (30)

- When the external ear of the left side is much affected and the ear is painful, hot, inflamed, with greenish-yellow discharge. *Puls.* (34)

- In case of violent intolerable pain in the ears with high irritability in children; the cheeks are red and the patient is restless; the symptoms are worse at night and from cold. *Cham.* (15)

## 76. EARS, NOISES IN THE

See EARS, HUMMING IN THE

## 77. ECZEMA

- For a dry, red, itchy eczema on the hands, wrists, often with multiple vesicle formation, irritation and tingling, worse at night and in damp weather, and better from heat. *Rhus-t.* (35)

- When with much itching, uncontrollable desire to scratch, which results in burning and soreness of the skin, worse at night, by heat of bed and bathing. *Sulph.* (39)

## 78. EPISTAXIS *(Nosebleed)*

- In case of severe nosebleed, generally due to concussion of brain from a fall, a blow, or excessive bodily exertion or shock, preceded by heat and itching of the nose, and the blood is dark bed fluid. **Arn.** (7)

- When in children from an unknown cause; blood bright red, which clots easily. **Ferr-p.** (20)

- Persistent in old people, when the blood is passive, profuse and non-coagulable. **Carb-v.** (14)

- For nosebleed in place of menses, or when the nose bleeds every morning and the blood is bright red. **Bry.** (11)

- When the blood is bright red and flows in gushes. **Ipec.** (25)

- For bleeding after being overheated, or in sanguine persons, with fever, strong pulsation of arteries of the sides of head (temples) and neck, and full hurried pulse. **Acon.** (1)

- When with flushed face, throbbing temples and congestion to head; profuse discharge of bright red blood. **Bell.** (9) *in alternation with* **Ferr-p.** (20)

- In females from suppressed or scanty monthly discharge. **Puls.** (34)

- If it arises from bodily exertion, or from lifting a heavy weight. **Rhus-t.** (35)

- When the patient is greatly agitated, restless, anxious and prostrated. **Ars.** (8)

**Note :** Persons subject to epistaxis should lead a temperate life, with moderate and regular exercise, a nourishing diet, avoiding stimulants, and should make a free use of cold water, especially about neck.

## 79. ERYSIPELAS *(Contagious Skin Infection)*

- If there is considerable fever, with hot dry skin, thirst and great restlessness. **Acon.** (1)

- If there be much fever and bright redness of affected part, with throbbing pain. **Bell.** (9)

- When the puffy swelling becomes prominent or small watery pustules form in abundance and skin be purplish. **Apis** (6)

- In dangerous cases, where there is a tendency to gangrene, and relief is obtained from general heat. **Ars.** (8)

## 80. EXHAUSTION

- If after unusual exercise, with bruised feeling all over the body, as if beaten. **Arn.** (7)

- When there is prostration and collapse with thirst, and a dry, cold skin, usually after an acute illness or diarrhoea, especially in chilly persons of fastidious mental makeup. **Ars.** (8)

- If there is exhaustion and collapse but the skin is cold and damp. **Carb-v.** (14)

## 81. EYE TROUBLES

- If the eye is red and acutely inflamed, with intolerable pain, or great dread of light, due to removal of any foreign body, or when dust or charcoal powder falls into the eyes. **Acon.** (1) *in alternation with* **Arn.** (7)

- If the eyes are sensitive to light and are convulsively closed, and there is dryness. and redness of the white of eye, and pain around the eye, and in the head. **Bell.** (9) *in alternation with* **Ferr-p.** (20)

- When the eyelids are glued together with profuse suppuration, or when the ailment assumes a protracted character. **Hep.** (23) *to be followed by* **Merc.** (30)

- For inflammation of the eyes with oedematous swelling of eyelids. **Apis** (6)

- When the mucous discharge and tears are acrid, and the lids get stuck in the morning and there is photophobia, blurred vision, worse from reading and writing. **Euphr.** (19)

- For eye-strains, or blackeye due to overwork, constant reading or writing, with blurred vision, aching pain in the eyeballs, or when the eyes are hot, tired and extremely painful. **Ruta** (36)

- In case of eye-strain, with double, dim or impaired vision, soreness of eyeballs, heaviness of lids and squinting associated with fatigue. **Gels.** (21)

- For aches and fatigue, often associated with inflammation due to infection. **Led.** (27)

- In case of inflammation without secretion of pus, burning with sensation as if grains of sand were under the eyelids. **Ferr-p.** (20)

- When the eyes discharge profuse bland yellowish pus, especially in open air and agglutinises the lids; or if the pains are of a pressive or shooting character. **Puls.** (34)

- When the troubles arise from a cold, and the mucus is of an acrid, corroding character and the pain is burning with dread of light. **Ars.** (8)

- If there is a sensation of sand under the eyelids or cutting pains, with itching and shooting. **Merc.** (30)

**Note :** In case of a foreign body, do not rub or press the eyes. Try gently to flush out the speck or foreign body with an eyewash of *Calendula* φ (one-half spoon of tincture into one cup of plain water).

*See also* **CONJUNCTIVITIS.**

## 82. EYELIDS, INFLAMMATION OF *(Blepharitis)*

- When the eyelids are swollen, hard and red, with heat, burning, dryness, pain and restlessness. **Acon.** (1)

- If the external surface or margins are much inflamed, or the margins are turned upwards. **Bell.** (9)

- If there are ulcers in the margins, with shooting, burning pains and itching in the eyes. **Merc.** (30)

- When the lids are swollen and painful, or to promote suppuration after matter has formed. **Hep.** (23)

- In case of ptosis (drooped or falling eyelids), when there is weakness, often associated with double vision, giddiness and pain in the eyeballs. **Gels.** (21)

- If there is much secretion of mucus with appearance of styes (small red swellings on eyelids) and much inflammatory redness of the lids. **Puls.** (34)

- If the lower lids are particularly swollen and the patient feels much heat, but is totally thirstless. **Apis.** (6)

- In case of recurrent, untidy-looking styes when the eyes are very red.   *Sulph.* (39)

## 83. FACE FLUSHED

- When with heat and throbbing.   *Bell.* (9)
- When due to exertion or with a slight rise in temperature.   *Ferr-p.* (20)

## 84. FACEACHE

- If there is great heat in the face, which is extremely red, with restlessness and irritation.   *Acon.* (1)
- In case of violent burning or tearing pain, worse at night, especially after midnight, with great restlessness and prostration (loss of strength).   *Ars.* (8)
- For darting pain under the eye, running mainly along the right cheek-bone, worse by slightest movement, noise, jar, warmth of bed, or a current of air.   *Bell.* (9)
- In case of violent rending and darting pains, running principally in the left side of the face and extending to the ear, sides of head, temples, nose and teeth.   *Colo.* (17)
- When the eyes are involved, or the pains increase with the day and decline towards evening.   *Spig.* (37)
- If there are drawing or jerking pains, worse by thinking, or cold air, or after eating.   *Nux-v.* (31)
- When the pains are worse at night, or with swelling of the cheeks.   *Merc.* (30)

EYELIDS, INFLAMMATION                    FACEACHE

## 85. FAINTING *(Syncope)*

- In case of fainting as soon as the patient sits up from a recumbent position, or due to fright, emotional excitement, or severe pain. ***Acon.*** (1)

- In case of fainting after sleep, while yet in bed or after rising in the morning. ***Carb-v.*** (14)

- If from severe pain or great excitability, or due to dentition, with dizziness, dimness of sight, hardness of hearing, sensation of qualmishness and flatness in the pit of the stomach. ***Cham.*** (15)

- If in the morning on rising, or after a meal, or from sight of blood, or from strong odour, or if fainting occurs in persons debilitated by excessive study, or sedentary habits. ***Nux-v.*** (31)

- In case of fainting from anger. ***Verat.*** (40)

- When due to fright, with dizziness and vertigo. ***Gels.*** (21)

- If due to loss of sleep, or when riding in a carriage, rail-road or motor-car, sea-boat, etc. ***Cocc.*** (16)

## 86. FATIGUE

- In case of fatigue of muscular origin, with aching, bruised pain and exhaustion, caused by any labour or physical exertion in walking, cycling, rowing, etc. ***Arn.*** (7)

- If from lifting or carrying heavy weights or loads. ***Rhus-t.*** (35)

COMMON AILMENTS AND THEIR REMEDIES 63

- When caused due to excessive studies, night-watching, and is accompanied with spasm, pain and weariness, and often, a trembling sensation and weakness of the legs. *Nux-v.* (31)

- If there is extreme exhaustion, poor circulation and cold clammy sweating, with cold extremities. *Carb-v.* (14)

- When associated with great restlessness and inability to relax; the patient is exhausted, cold, chilly, especially after an attack of flu, or generally in run-down subjects. *Ars.* (8)

## 87. FEAR, PANIC, ETC.

- In case of sudden fear, particularly the fear of death, or "out of blue", desperate, impatient, restless and inappeasable; fear of crowds, crossing a road, etc. *Acon.* (1)

- In case of sudden uncontrollable fear, especially when alone, associated with nausea, restlessness, intolerable anguish and great prostration; fears that his disease is incurable. *Ars.* (8)

- When the patient is paralysed with fear, knees quiver, trembles all over, wants to be held firmly to control the shaking, especially before an ordeal; examination fear. *Gels.* (21)

- For fear of downward motion, with great anxiety; when laying the baby on a couch or in the crib, it cries and clings to the nurse. *Bor.* (10)

FATIGUE	FEAR, PANIC, ETC.

## 88. FEVERS

- When the skin is hot and dry, face red or pale on rising, alternating chills and flushes, intense thirst for large quantities of cold water, great restlessness, and tossing about. **Acon.** (1)
- When the skin is burning hot, face and eyes red, with throbbing headache, confusion, and severe chilliness; or when the head head is fiery hot, carotids (neck arteries) throbbing and feet cold, or when there is high fever with glandular involvement. **Bell.** (9) *in alternation with* **Ferr-p.** (20)
- When attended with heaviness in head, or headache and cough, yellow-coated tongue, constipation, intense stitching pain in chest and head on coughing, great thirst; complaints are worse from movement. **Bry.** (11)
- When attended with chill, without thirst; chills running up and down the spine; head and eyes heavy and painful; the patient is dull, drowsy and dizzy. **Gels.** (21)
- In case of intermittent fever, with nausea, chill and thirst; body hot, extremities cold. **Ipec.** (25)
- When the fever is followed by exposure to cold and damp, or is attended with diarrhoea, great weakness, restlessness and prostration. **Rhus-t.** (35)
- When the fever is severe and prolonged, and is accompanied with anguish, great heat, shivering, loss of strength, and the patient takes frequent sips of water and finds relief from heat. **Ars.** (8)
- When there is hoarseness, with rattling of mucus in the windpipe, or if there is shivering with internal heat. **Cham.** (15)
- If the fever is accompanied with much sneezing, profuse discharge of mucus from

the nose, hoarseness and soreness in the throat and profuse foul perspiration which does not abate; the patient cannot tolerate both extremes of heat and cold. **Merc. (30)**

- When fever is associated with acute coryza and accompanie with heaviness of head, general aching of limbs, great chilliness and stuffy nose. **Nux-v. (31)**

- When the fever is caused due to cold and damp, with pain. **Rhus-t. (35)**

**Note :** In high fever, sponging the face and forehead with cold water will reduce the temperature and make the patient comfortable. But if it persists or continues to rise in spite of administering the indicated homoeopathic remedies, call in the physician immediately.

## 89. FITS, CONVULSIONS, SPASMS

- When the fit is caused as the result of fright. **Acon. (1)**

- When associated with drowsiness after vomiting and/or purging, pupils large and fixed (half open), thumb and teeth clenched. **Aethuja (2)**

- When the fits get worse by hot bath, or heat in any form with stiffness of neck muscles and sudden shrill cry. **Apis (6)**

- In case of sudden onset of a fit, when connected with disturbances of the brain and derangement of nervous system, with burning skin, big staring pupils, hot or flushed face, or inflammation of the brain, violent movements, worse from light and least jar. **Bell. (9)**

- In case of involuntary movements of the head, great restlessness and jerking of the limbs, caused by anger, or teething; thumbs

- clenched in palms, spasmodic twitching of the eyelids and muscles of the face, paleness of one cheek and redness of the other; or when there is much acidity of stomach. **Cham.** (15)

- When the fit is especially brought on by exposure to the heat of the sun; the head is hot and congested, face dusky and pupils small. **Glon.** (22)

- When the brain is the seat of affection and there is spasm of the throat and threatened suffocation. **Gels.** (21) *in alternation with* **Bell.** (9)

- If occasioned by indigestible food, or overloading stomach or if there is nausea, vomiting or diarrhoea. **Ipec.** (25)

- To remove weakness after fits or convulsions. **Carb-v.** (14)

## 90. FLATULENCE *(Excessive Gas in Abdomen)*

- When arising from eating starchy, rich, fatty foods, pastries, etc. **Puls.** (34)

- If there is abundant flatulence, or if it is worse after eating and drinking, or when from over, indulgence in diet, with sour, bitter eructations or when associated with constipation, constricting pain. **Nux-v.** (31)

- When there is distension of upper abdomen with pain and windy belchings, which get relieved for a time. **Carb-v.** (14)

- In case of excessive accumulation of wind in the lower abdomen, especially after eating bread, beans, cabbage; eating so little causes fullness which is somewhat relieved by passing loud noisy flatus. **Lyco.** (28)

- In case of flatulence of infants, better after bringing up winds and associated with irritability.  **Cham.** (15)

## 91. FLU : See INFLUENZA.

## 92. FOOD POISONING : See POISONING.

## 93. FRACTURES
- When they are slow to heal.  **Calc-p.** (12)

## 94. GIDDINESS : See VERTIGO.

## 95. GLAUCOMA *(Eye disease with intense pressure within eyeballs and progressive dimness of vision)*

- In the acute form of glaucoma with great restlessness and anxiety.  **Acon.** (1)
- When the onset is violent and acute with inflammation, dryness and photophobia.  **Bell.** (9)
- If tension within eyeballs (Intraocular tension) is raised and there is intense soreness, watering and Photophobia (intolerance of light).  **Bry.** (11)
- When the eyes feel bruised and under pressure with double, dim or misty vision.  **Gels.** (21)
- When the eyeballs feel too large and pulled back into the head, sometimes accompanying sharp, shooting and sticking pains, palpitation of heart, and the symptoms are worse from movement and at night.  **Spig.** (37)

## 96. GOUT
- In acute cases with febrile symptoms and

- great sensibility to touch, or throbbing in the foot, especially at commencement, and in Plethoric (full-blooded) subjects. **Acon.** (1)
- In wandering gout, with shifting pain, or at the commencement when the joint has become attacked, and the pain is worse by rising from a seat or lying down. **Puls.** (34) *in alternation with* **Acon.** (1)
- When the attacks are traceable to spirituous liquors and other stimulants or luxurious living, with indigestion or irregular action of bowels, or if there is a sensation of numbness in the affected parts. **Nux-v.** (31)
- In case of gout implicating the chest, or with bilious symptoms and if the pains are aggravated by movement or if there is red, hot swelling, with shooting pains. **Bry.** (11)
- When the affected parts feel painfully bruised and are extremely sensitive to touch. **Arn.** (7)
- When the disease starts in the lower extremities and travels upwards, the pain is worse from warmth and better by cold applications. **Led.** (27)
- When the affected joint is red, hot, swollen and unbearably tender, sensitive to the least touch, jar or movement and better from cold compresses and exposure to cool air. **Bell.** (9)

## 97. GUMBOILS

- In case of heat, pain and swelling, with anxiety and great restlessness. **Acon.** (1)
- If there is great heat, inflammation, throbbing pain, and the part is fiery red and tender to touch. **Bell.** (9)

- For considerable throbbing, pain and salivation. **Merc. (30)**
- To promote suppuration (pus) when matter has formed. **Hep. (23)**

## 98. GUMS— BLEEDING, PAINFUL, ULCERATED

- When the gums bleed profusely after tooth extraction. Helpful generally for shock and weakness. **Arn. (7)**
- In case of painful and swollen gums after tooth extraction. **Hyper. (24)** *in alternation with* **Arn. (7)**
- If the gums bleed much or if they are sore and ulcerated. **Carb-v. (14)**
- When the teeth are loose and ready to fall out, the gums are fungous, livid and ulcerated, with foul breath and metallic taste. **Merc. (30)**
- In case of bleeding, with putrid and painful swelling of the gums. **Nux-v. (31)**
- When there is oozing of bright red blood from gums for any reason. **Phos. (32)**

**Note :** Rinse the mouth with *Calendula lotion* (10 drops of *Calundula* φ in a teacupful of boiled and cooled water).

## 99. HAEMORRHAGE *(Bleeding)*

- When the haemorrhage follows a fall, strain, mis-step, overexertion or other mechanical injuries (to prevent both bleeding and shock). **Arn. (7)** *in alternation with* **Acon. (1)**
- If there is a steady oozing of dark blood with sudden collapse, cold breath, coldness of limbs, cold sweat and air hunger. **Carb-v. (14)**

- In case of gushes of bright red arterial blood coming from any orifice, especially the nose, or the lungs, with severe nausea, cold sweat, weak pulse and gasping for breath.
  **Ipec.** (25)
  *in alternation with*
  **Ferr-p.** (20)

- When the blood is of cherry red colour and accompanied with great excitement, panic, anguish, palpitation, thirst for cold water and full hurried pulse.
  **Acon.** (1)

- If there is great restlessness, anxiety and marked loss of strength.
  **Ars.** (8)

- When the blood is bright red and hot, and clots easily and accompanies congestion in the head, red and hot face, full and bounding pulse.
  **Bell.** (9)
  *in alternation with*
  **Ferr-p.** (20)

- When there is bleeding every morning, and blood is dark and fluid, with nausea, and aggravation of all symptoms by movement and better from rest.
  **Bry.** (11)

- When there is oozing of bright red blood.
  **Phos.** (32)

- In case of bleeding for any reason and from any outlet of the body, when the blood is bright red, clots readily and flows profusely.
  **Ferr-p.** (20)

- In case of bleeding from intestines, accompanied with collapse, cold sweat on face and air hunger.
  **Verat.** (40)

- For nasal haemorrhage in females with scanty monthly discharge.
  **Puls.** (34)

Note : In case of bleeding gum, place a plug of cotton wool or thin gauze strip soaked in *Calendula* ϕ on the gum and let it remain there until the bleeding stops. In case of external haemorrhage, from a cut or injury, press the sterile gauze (or the cleanest material available) firmly over the wound. When the bleeding has stopped, clean the part with *Calendula* mixing it with water in the ratio of 1:3. Dress bandage firmly on the wound and take the patient to a doctor; if necessary, and administer any of the aforementioned remedies as per indications.

## 100. HAEMORRHOIDS: See PILES.

## 101. HALITOSIS: See BAD BREATH

## 102. HEADACHE

- In case of a sudden violent headache, usually due to dry, cold winds, with congestion in head, hemicrania (one-side headache), great restlessness, anxiety and thirst and sensation as if skull contents would be forced out through forehead, throbbing in temples better by rest and worse by noise and movement. *Acon.* (1)

- For bursting headache, violent throbbing and shooting, face red and hot, dilated pupils, worse with least jar, noise, motion, stooping, coughing, or light, and better by wrapping the head warmly and lying straight on the back. *Bell.* (9)

- For bursting or splitting headache, worse from any motion, stooping, opening or moving the eyes and coughing, and better during rest. *Bry.* (11)

- When the pain is in the right side and back of head, which extends to shoulders and is associated with heavy eyelids and limbs, dim or blurred vision, giddiness and general malaise, worse with heat of sun, noise, light, movement and tobacco-smoking and better by passing profuse urine and sitting by reclining the head on high pillow. *Gels.* (21)

- In case of the waves of terrible bursting,

throbbing pain, with increased urination, upward surging of hot blood, usually as a result of exposure to heat of sun, better for cold air, sleep and lying down with head high.　　　　　　　　　　　　　　　　*Glon.* (23)

- In case of sick headache, with retching and little vomiting.　　　　　　　　　　　*Cocc.* (16)

- If arising from a fall or blow, an injury (either recent or old) or fatigue, and there is bruise-like pain in the head (mainly forehead), worse by any movement.　　*Arn.* (7)

- For splitting headache, with a feeling as if a nail were driven into the skull, with nausea and sour vomiting, or when there are heaviness in the forehead and stuffiness of nose, or as a result of over-indulgence in foods or alcoholic beverages, or catarrhal conditions, i.e., with inflammatory discharges from upper respiratory tract, worse after meals and stooping, in the morning on waking, after alcohol and in the open air, and better in warmth, on lying down and covering the head.　*Nux-v.* (31)

- When the pain is relieved by bending the head backwards.　　　　　　　　　　　*Hyper.* (24)

- In case of catarrh, i.e., inflammation of mucous membranes with discharge, when the headache arises from a slightest chill, or from suppression of perspiration, or when from anger or passion.　　　　*Cham.* (15)

- When the headache is accompanied by frequent sneezing and much running of the nose, or chilliness, with pain in the limbs.　*Merc.* (30)

- In case of headache with nausea and vomiting.　　　　　　　　　　　　　　　　*Ipec.* (25)

- When the headache is periodic, throbbing and variable, and is connected with the derangement or acidity of the stomach, or from rich starchy foods, fat meats, pastries, etc., and is better from cool applications, open air and slow walking and worse for looking up and lying down. **Puls.** (34)
- When with painful, watering eyes and inability to bear light. **Euphr.** (19)
- In case of headache with vertigo, in anaemic subjects. **Calc-p.** (12)

## 103. HEART ATTACK

- For acute attacks with severe pain about the heart, worse for activity, with great restlessness and fear of death. **Acon.** (1) *in alternation with* **Arn.** (7)
- In case of senile (old age) heart disease when the ankles become blue and swollen and the heart feels constricted. **Lach.** (26)
- When the attacks accompany palpitation of heart with pain in the chest and back and are worse from motion. **Spig.** (37)
- In case of thin, chilly, over-anxious and fearful subjects who are uncertain of future, and generally unable to share and express their underlying fears and feeling. **Ars.** (8)
- In case of high-pitched, over-controlled, ambitious executives; short-tempered subjects of sedentary (sitting) habits. **Nux-v.** (31)

## 104. HEARTBURN *(Burning of food pipe by acidity)*

- If occasioned by excessive in wine or other

- spirituous liquors, or when from weakness of stomach, with nausea after eating, vomiting of food, or periodical vomiting after eating. **Nux-v. (31)**
- For constant burning and belching of wind. **Carb-v. (14)**
- When there is strong desire to vomit, or in case of chronic vomiting, or vomiting from over-loading the stomach with rich, fat food. **Puls. (34)**
- When occurring at summer time, or in damp and warm weather, as a result of dyspepsia (indigestion). **Bry. (11)**

## 105. HEART, PAIN ABOUT: See ANGINA PECTORIS

## 106. HEART, PALPITATION OF

- When due to fear or excitement, with anxiety, coldness, numbness in the lower extremities, or a sensation as if the heart had ceased to beat; short, hurried breathing, hot and flushed face, fainting. **Acon. (1)**
- For oppression, tremor, palpitation extending to the neck and head, congested face. **Bell. (9)**
- In case of nervous palpitation, with a feeling that the muscles are not obeying the will. **Gels. (21)**
- For palpitation with pain about the heart, particularly when the palpitation is violent, visible and audible, and is worse from least motion and bending forward. **Spig. (37)**
- When from anger, excitement or passion, and the pain is intolerable. **Cham. (15)**

- For hysterical symptoms and in females suffering from delayed periods, or nervousness, when the palpitation is very violent, or occurs in the evening. **Puls. (34)**
- If it occurs in robust persons, or in the morning, usually associated with indigestion, constipation and irritability. **Nux-v. (31)**

## 107. HERPES: See SHINGLES

## 108. HICCOUGH

- If from taking cold drinks, or during fever. **Ars. (8)**
- In case of very obstinate type of hiccough, with persistent soreness in the chest. **Mag-p. (29)**
- When due to digestive disturbances, or alcoholic beverages, or if occuring before meals. **Nux-v. (31)**
- If caused by taking hot drinks, or after a spell of vomiting. **Verat. (40)**
- When hiccough is violent, with red face. **Bell. (9)**
- When hiccough is worse from drinking water. **Merc. (30)**

## 109. HIGH BLOOD PRESSURE

See BLOOD PRESSURE, HIGH

## 110. HOARSENESS

- For dryness, roughness and sensation of fullness in the throat, with feverishness. **Acon. (1)**
- When with a sense of constriction and rawness of the throat. **Bell. (9)**

- In case of severe cold, with much chilliness, thick discharge from the nostrils, tickling and burning in the throat, sneezing, shivering, disposition to perspire and aggravation of symptoms in the evening. **Merc.** (30)

- For weak and hoarse voice, wheezing breathing, in old cases, when there is much roughness and soreness in the chest or the hoarseness follow cold damp weather. **Hep.** (23)

- For chronic hoarseness which is worse in damp weather, and in the evening; aphonia (loss of voice). **Carb-v.** (14)

- In case of violent catarrh (inflammation with discharge) with great hoarseness, or with cough and dryness in the throat, or when the larynx or chest feels rough and sore and the patient is having a consumptive tendency. **Phos.** (32)

- When from overstraining the voice. **Arn.** (7) *in alternation with* **Calc-p.** (12)

- In recent cases, when the complaints arise from a chill, with much phlegm, or rattling of mucus, the spot in the throat feeling sore wherefrom mucus is detached. **Cham.** (15)

- If there is a stuffy feeling in the head, or there is a dry, rough, exhaustive cough. **Nux-v.** (31)

## 111. HOOPING COUGH: *See WHOOPING COUGH*

## 112. HYPERTENSION: *See BLOOD PRESSURE, HIGH*

## 113. HYPOTENSION: *See BLOOD PRESSURE, LOW*

## 114. INDIGESTION

- When arising from a sedentary (sitting or motionless) life, hot weather, or overheating, and there is weight-like pain in the stomach immediately after eating, sometimes with bilious vomiting, nausea, bitter taste and frontal headache. **Bry (11).**

- For distension of gas, flatulence and acidity, nausea with sour acid taste, sour belchings, when the simple food does not agree and causes gas in the abdomen and pain in the abdominal epigastrium (stomach). **Carb-v. (14)**

- If due to a sedentary life, prolonged watching, eating or drinking in excess, excessive study or mental exertion, taking coffee, cold food, alebeer, wine, other spirituous liquors or tobacco and is accompanied by nausea and vomiting, heartburn, sour and bitter taste, bitter belching, pain in the abdomen few hours after eating, and frequent urging for stools with rumbling and flatulence. **Nux-v. (31)**

- If it arises from an injury blow, or a fall, or fatigue. **Arn. (7)**

- For indigestion in weak patients, delayed digestion, empty all gone sensation, sleepy after meals, especially dinner, flatulence (gas) with noisy rumblings and nausea, sluggish bowels, sandy urine and craving for sweet things. **Lyco. (28)**

- For simple retching or nausea and easy vomiting, but with great force, from gastric derangements, without inflammation of the stomach, or any grave affection of the mucous membrane. **Ipec. (25)**

- For chronic indigestion when nearly all kinds of food disagree. Ill-effects of Mercurial poisoning. **Hep. (23)**

- In case of indigestion of weak, exhausted and chilly subjects who lack appetite and suffer from burning or excessive pain in the stomach, nausea, vomiting and diarrhoea, better for heat, in general, except the head symptoms which are relieved by cold. **Ars.** (8)

- When arising from prolonged watching, eating in excess, especially rich foods, butter, fat, meat, hot or spoiled food and tobacco, with loss of taste, thirstlessness, spasmodic pains, pressure in the stomach with vomiting or rumbling, mucous or watery diarrhoea, white-coated tongue, thirstlessness worse in the evening. **Puls.** (34)

- In case of chronic indigestion with sour, offensive belchings, flatulence, constipation or piles with itching anus, and excessive drinking. **Sulph.** (39) *to be followed by* **Nux-v.** (31)

- When accompanied with gastritis (inflammation of inner lining of stomach), pain, swelling and tenderness of the stomach, hot flushed face, vomiting of undigested food, undigested stools. **Ferr-p.** (20)

- When the complaints are caused by anger or indignation, and are accompanied by colic and diarrhoea, cutting or griping pains, which are relieved by hard pressure and bending double. **Colo.** (17)

- When indigestion is caused due to anger or passion. **Cham.** (15)

- If from fright or anxiety. **Acon.** (1)

## 115. INFLAMMATION

- In the first stage of all inflammations. **Ferr-p.** (20) *in alternation with* **Bell.** (9)

## 116. INFLUENZA (Flu)

- For the premonitory chill, rigors and fever, particularly in children before the disease is fully developed, to abort attack. **Acon.** (1)

- For the loss of muscular power, fever or feverishness, fatigue, weakness and general aching and soreness of the whole body, dullness, drowsiness and dizziness and when the chills run up and down the spine, watering eyes and frequent sneezing; thirstlessness. **Gels.** (21)

- In case of epidemic influenza, with profuse acid discharge from nose, sneezing, sometimes diarrhoea, burning, pains, exhaustion, weakness and prostration, and great thirst for frequent sips of water, better for warmth in general. **Ars.** (8)

- When the catarrhal symptoms are priminent, the nose is swollen and there is much bad smelling perspiration. **Merc.** (30)

- For dizziness and subsequent debility when the patient is constipated, irritable, chilly, and has general aching and pains in the body, particularly in the back region. **Nux-v.** (31)

- When the limbs are heavy and there are dry cough, fever, frontal headache, pain in the whole body, dryness of lips and tongue, and aggravation from least jar or movement. **Bry.** (11)

- If accompanied with small and rapid pulse, dry hot skin, dryness of tongue, heat and pain in the head, and throbbing in temples. **Bell.** (9) *in alternation with* **Ferr-p.** (20)

- For the debility remaining after the attack, or for the bronchial symptoms. **Phos.** (32)

- For weakness resulting after influenza, to tone up the vitality. **Calc-p.** (12)

## 117. INJURIES: See WOUNDS.

## 118. INSECT STINGS: See BITES AND STINGS

## 119. INSOMNIA: See SLEEPLESSNESS

## 120. IRRITABILITY

- When from jealousy, fright, anger or grief. **Apis** (6)
- In case of teething children crying for nothing. **Cham.** (15)
- In ill-tempered persons. **Bry.** (11)
- If due to overwork, or when caused due to coffee, alcoholic beverages, cigarettes and night-watching. **Nux-v.** (31)

## 121. ITCHING

- For severe itching with dryness, burning and redness of the skin, worse in the evening, after bathing and in the warmth of bed; scratching is pleasurable, but results in soreness and burning. **Sulph.** (39)
- For feverish heat, redness of the skin, thirst and when the symptoms are worse at night. **Acon.** (1)
- For itching and redness with swelling and tingling, worse during rest. **Rhus-t.** (35)
- When with burning, or with an eruption emitting small drops of watery fluid, better from general warmth. **Ars.** (8)
- When itching is relieved by cold bathing or cold applications. **Led.** (27)
- When itching is worse at night for the heat of bed, with thirstlessness. **Puls.** (34)
- In case of recurrent eruptions, which ooze, and are chronically sore and irritating. **Merc.** (30)

## 122. JAUNDICE

- In case of high fever, or where there is much tenderness about the region of liver. **Acon.** (1)
- When the complaint arises from the abuse of spirituous liquors, or in persons of sedentary (idle) habits, with much constipation. **Nux-v.** (31)
- When arising from anger or passion, or if occasioned by a chill, with great irritability and restlessness. **Cham.** (15)
- When the inflammatory symptoms have modified. **Merc.** (30)

## 123. JOINTS, PAINFUL

- If due to strenuous straining, excessive bodily exertion, or rheumatic conditions, when there is stiffness and the pains are worse on rising, during rest, cold and damp, and better from continued motion and heat. **Rhus-t.** (35)
- When the serous membranes are affected; the joints are swollen and pains are worse from motion, heat or jar, and better with rest and pressure. **Bry.** (11)
- In case of arthritis and rheumatism of the hip and large joints, or if the pain is felt more in periosteum (covering) of bones and the patient feels better in warm damp weather. **Ruta** (36)
- When the knees crack a lot and the pains are arthritic and of shifting nature, worse from heat and better for walking in cool weather. **Puls.** (34)

## 124. LACHRYMATION *(Watering of eyes)*

- When due to fall or injury to head, or a foreign body in the eye. **Arn.** (7)

- When resulting from coryza (nasal cold), with much burning in the eyes, and hot excoriating (corroding) discharge. **Ars.** (8)

- In case of profuse bland discharge from the eyes, and corroding watery discharge from the nose, with sneezing. **All-c.** (3)

- When there is profuse acrid watery discharge from the eyes and bland discharge from the nose with margins of lids red, swollen and burning. **Euphr.** (19)

- When the patient weeps, when detailing her ailments. **Puls.** (34)

## 125. LARYNGITIS *(Inflammation of larynx)*

- In case of acute laryngitis due to cold winds or draughts, accompanied with dry croupy cough, fever, chill, dryness of skin, hoarseness, great restlessness and anxiety. **Acon.** (1)

- When the larynx feels sore and swollen and there is irritating cough, and the complaints are usually caused due to shock or fear. **Arn.** (7)

- In case of high temperature, a red flushed face, dilated pupils, sweating and pain in throat with a dry barking cough. **Bell.** (9)

- For hoarseness due to cold dry winds or draughts, worse in the morning, and better with warmth; hoarseness of singers and public speakers. **Hep.** (23)

- In case of a sore dryness in the larynx with a rough voice, dry cough, painful talking and hoarseness, worse in the evening. **Phos.** (32)

- For painless hoarseness, usually caused by exposure to damp cold air, worse in the evening, cold perspiration with chilliness. **Carb-v.** (14)

## 126. LEUCORRHOEA *(Whites)*

- When the discharge is thick and creamy, acrid, burning and excoriating, associated with chilliness and depressive tenderness. **Puls.** (34)
- In case of thick, greenish and very corrosive discharge worse at night. **Merc.** (30)
- For leucorrhoea in place of menses. **Cocc.** (16)
- When the discharge is like the white of an egg, clear and copious, feels hot and occurs in the middle of the cycles usually, is painless, with associated general anxiety and tension. **Bor.** (10)
- In obstinate cases, with burning in palms and soles, usually for those who eat little and drink more. **Sulph.** (39)

## 127. LIGAMENTS/TENDONS, PAINFUL *(Fibrous bands connecting bones/ends of muscles joining a bone)*

- If the pains are due to overexertion of the body and they are worse in cold and during rest and better stretching the limbs. **Rhus-t.** (35)
- When due to overstraining of flexor tendons, which are worse on stretching limbs. **Ruta** (36)

## 128. LIGHT INTOLERABLE *(Photophobia)*

- When with watering, stinging eyes. **Euphr.** (19)
- When the eyes are red and pupils contracted. **Bell.** (9)

## 129. LIPS, DRY

- When with excessive thirst and constipation. **Bry.** (11)

## 130. LUMBAGO *(Backache)*

- If the pain is sharp, as if beaten or sprained and suddenly brought on by exposure to dry cold winds and accompanies much fever, and restlessness. **Acon.** (1)
- If there is bruise-like pain, usually caused by a blow, fall, external injury or overlifting, or muscular strain. **Arn.** (7)
- If due to muscular strain, or from getting wet, especially when overheated, or due to suppressed perspiration, with increase of pain during rest and at night, on first moving the affected part, or on first getting up in the morning, better during continued motion. **Rhus-t.** (35)
- When the pains are severe and compel the patient to walk in a stooping posture, and are worse on movement, or draught of cold air. **Bry.** (11)
- When the pains are deep-seated, throbbing and cause heaviness, gnawing or stiffness. **Bell.** (9)
- If the back feels fatigued or bruised, or if there be constipation, or symptoms of indigestion. **Nux-v.** (31)
- For acute inflammatory pains in the loins. **Ferr-p.** (20)
  *in alternation with*
  **Mag-p.** (29)
- In case of severe pains on bending, inability to straighten, rheumatic pains in joints with cold and numb feeling and when the symptoms are worse from cold and change of weather. **Calc-p.** (12)

## 131. LUNGS, INFLAMMATION OF *(Pneumonia)*

- Whenever inflammatory symptoms run high and the secretory functions are suspended. **Acon.** (1)

- For laboured, short and rapid breathing, with stitching and burning pains in the sides; painful dry cough, worse on inspiration and movement. **Bry. (11)**

- In case of severe sticking pain in the chest, excited or increased by breathing; short, dry cough with rust-coloured sputa. **Phos. (32)**

- When the breathing is greatly suppressed and the cough is attended with much rattling of mucus in the chest, which cannot be raised. **Ant-t. (5)**

- In tedious cases, with extreme loss of strength, painfully oppressed breathing, better by warmth, in general. **Ars. (8)**

- When the prominent symptoms have abated or yielded to other remedies. **Sulph. (39)**

## 132. MASTITIS *(Inflammation of breasts)*

- When the whole breast is hard, painful and tense, with stitching pains and occasional headache. **Bry. (11)**

- When the breast is hot with streaks radiating red, pulsating pains, worse from movement, touch or jar. **Bell. (9)**

- When there is possibility of abscess formation. **Merc. (30)**

- When the abscess has developed. **Hep. (23)**

- When the pain is burning and usually associated with overlying skin disease. **Sulph. (39)**

## 133. MEASLES

- In the early stages, when there is high fever, full pulse, dry cough, constipation,

- restlessness, sleeplessness, inflammation of eyes, great thirst and tossing-about in agony.  *Acon.* (1)

- In case of delirium, sore throat, severe pain in head, or great intolerance of light.  *Bell.* (9)

- For the imperfectly developed or suppressed eruption, stitching pain in the chest, difficulty in breathing and dry hacking cough; symptoms worse on movement and the least jar.  *Bry.* (11)

- When the skin is warm, hot and burning, throat painful and swollen, intolerance of heat or warmth (though the least cold draught or cool air is intolerable).  *Ferr-p.* (20)

- In case of high fever, suppressed eruptions, thirst, headache, constipation, delirium, prostration, dry tongue and convulsions.  *Gels.* (21)

- When the catarrhal symptoms are mainly confined to nose and eyes and the eyes are very sore, with moderate temperature, photophobia (allergy to light).  *Euphr.* (19)

- When the disease is complicated with bad congestive bronchitis.  *Ant-t.* (5)

- In case of cough which is worse in the evening, with yellow catarrhal discharge from the nose and throat, sometimes, diarrhoea, intestinal and stomach upsets, restlessness and irritability, thirstlessnes.  *Puls.* (34)

- In the later stages, when there is hoarse and (suffocative) cough, worse with cold and draught of cool air.  *Hep.* (23)

- When the eruptions has completed its normal course.  *Sulph.* (39)

- When the skin symptoms have cleared up and fever has abated, to tone up vitality.  *Calc-p.* (12)

**MEASLES**

## 134. MENOPAUSE: See CHANGE OF LIFE

## 135. MENORRHAGIA: See MENSES, EXCESSIVE

## 136. MENSES ABSENT: See AMENORRHOEA

## 137. MENSES DELAYED: See AMENORRHOEA

## 138. MENSES EXCESSIVE *(Spating; Menorrhagia)*

- When in plethoric (full-blooded) subjects, with hot discharge, pressing downward with bright red blood. **Bell.** (9)
- When the discharge is profuse and continued and amounts to flooding. **Ipec.** (25)
- When the menses are too profuse and too frequent, worse at night and there is cramping pain in the lower abdomen. **Bor.** (10)
- When the flooding is associated with pain in the lower abdomen and back, and symptoms are always variable and changing. **Puls.** (34)
- When the heavy flow or flooding accompanies severe cramping pain; with passage of clots and flushes of heat, with anger and irritability. **Lach.** (26)
- In case of excessive flooding, with great restlessness and extreme prostration (loss of strength). **Ars.** (8)

## 139. MENSES PAINFUL *(Dysmenorrhoea)*

- When there is pressing, cutting, spasmodic and throbbing pain in the lower abdomen one day before the flow, the intestines feel forced through the vagina and the face is red. **Bell.** (9)

- In case of cutting and tearing pains in lower abdomen and back, loss of appetite with vomiting, chill, diarrhoea during menses, and scanty or profuse flow with clots. *Puls.* (34)

- When there is sharp cutting pain in the abdomen which is worse by every movement, every breath, with nausea to the point of fainting and vertigo, a fitful, scanty and irregular discharge. *Cocc.* (16)

- In case of spasmodic sharp pains in the lower abdomen and back, with heavy, besotted-looking face, congested eyes, painful discharge, great weakness, and when the muscles do not obey the will. *Gels.* (21)

- In case of painful menstruation, bright red flow, flushed face, quickened pulse, congestion of pelvic organs, with too profuse loss of blood. *Ferr-p.* (20)

- In case of spasmodic pains, cramps, labour-like bearing-down pains, menstrual colic, better by bending double or hard pressure. *Mag-p.* (29) *in alternation with* *Colo.* (17)

- If labour-like pain, with pressure from the small of back, or colic with tenderness of the abdomen, occurs or if the discharge is very dark-coloured, dirty with "clots" and the patient is irritable. *Cham.* (15)

- When the forcing pain predominates, or if there be nausea and fainting, or congestion of blood to head, giddiness, and great debility. *Nux-v.* (31)

- When the periods are irregular and the pain has a burning character. *Sulph.* (39)

- In anaemic subjects and girls at puberty. *Calc-p.* (12)

## 140. MENSES RETARDED: See AMENORRHOEA

## 141. MENSES SCANTY: See AMENORRHOEA

## 142. MENSES SUPPRESSED: See AMENORRHOEA

## 143. MILK-CRUST *(Hard crust in scalp of nursing infants)*

- If there is great irritation and the eruption bleeds easily. **Merc.** (30)
- In obstinate cases. **Sulph.** (39)

## 144. MORNING SICKNESS *(Nausea and Vomiting, especially in Pregnancy)*

- When it gets worse, while lying down with nausea. **Ipec.** (25)
- When retching and nausea are prominent, but vomiting is not marked. **Nux-v.** (31)

See also Pregnancy, Disorders of.

## 145. MOSQUITO BITES: See BITES AND STINGS

## 146. MOTION SICKNESS

- For nausea, vomiting and vertigo, salivation, or if there is a tendency to faint, while riding in a carriage, boat, car, or rail-road transport, worse from smell of food and better lying down. **Cocc.** (16)
- If associated with constipation, indigestion and splitting headache; mild sickness. **Nux-v.** (31)
- In case of air sickness when there is dread of downward motion. **Bor.** (10)
- If there is nausea, restlessness, especially in as seekness with relief by lying down. **Rhus-t.** (35)
- For extreme weakness and loss of strength after an attack. **Ars.** (8)

**Note :** *Nux vomica* should be taken before going on board a ship, preparing for sailing.

## 147. MOUTH, TASTE IN

- For strong metallic slimy taste with flow of saliva.    ***Cupr.*** (18)
- In case of bitter or sweetish metallic taste and coppery saliva.    ***Merc.*** (30)
- In case of bitter taste accompanied with constipation and thirst, gulping large quantities of cold water at long intervals.    ***Bry.*** (11)
- When the bread tastes bitter or when there is no taste at all.    ***Puls.*** (30)
- When there is great thirst and everything tastes bitter except water.    ***Acon.*** (1)

## 148. MUMPS *(Parotitis)*

- In acute early stages when there is fever, restlessness, thirst and pain.    ***Acon.*** (1)
- If the right side is prominently affected and there is much fever, pain, redness and swelling of parotid glands, worse by the least jar.    ***Bell.*** (9) *may be followed by* ***Merc.*** (30)
- When the left-sided glands are affected, with swelling and redness, worse from cold and damp weather.    ***Rhus-t.*** (35)
- For pus-forming and severe complications.    ***Hep.*** (23)
- When there is metastasis (transfer) of mumps to testicles or breasts.    ***Puls.*** (34)
- If the infection becomes a complication of the illness.    ***Sulph.*** (39)

## 149. MUSCULAR PAINS: *See PAINS*

## 150. MUSCULAR SORENESS

- If after a prolonged or strenuous exercise or being beaten, or incurring traumatic injury.  *Arn.* (7)
*in alternation with*
*Rhus-t.* (35)

## 151. NAUSEA *(Tendency to vomit)*

- For nausea and retching after eating and drinking, vomiting of blood, or little brown-black mucus mixed with blood or green mucus and great prostration (loss of strength).  *Ars.* (8)
- For nausea, vomiting and vertigo, while travelling by bus, car, rail or sea.  *Cocc.* (16)
- In case of constant and continued nausea with great flow of saliva, griping pain in intestines, clear tongue and marked prespiration, green or mucous vomit.  *Ipec.* (25)
- When the nausea and retching are brought on by indigestion and overeating, or after eating in the morning.  *Nux-v.* (31)

## 152. NECK, STIFF: See STIFF-NECK

## 153. NERVOUSNESS

- In case of weak head, difficulty in thinking, backache and when the patient imagines seeing faces in the dark.  *Phos.* (32)
- If the patient is irritable, loses temper at slightest things and everything goes wrong, with sleeplessness, nightmares, angry at everything, etc.  *Nux-v.* (31)
- In case of nervous pains, cramps and nervous twitchings.  *Mag-p.* (29)
- To improve the quality of blood and to promote assimilation of vital nutrients.  *Calc-p.* (12)

## 154. NETTLE-RASH: See URTICARIA

## 155. NEURALGIA *(Pain in nerves)*

- When with flushed, hot face. **Bell.** (9)
- For all sorts of neuralgic pains, cramps and spasms. **Mag-p.** (29)
- In case of inflammatory conditions, caused by chills, fevers, etc. **Ferr-p.** (20)
- When the pains are relieved by hard pressure. **Colo.** (17)

## 156. NIGHTMARE *(Oppressive and suffocative frightful dreams with immobility)*

- If accompanied with fever, palpitation of heart, or oppression of chest. **Acon.** (1)
- When with headache on waking, flushed face and irritation about the eyes. **Bell.** (9)
- If as a result of spirituous liquors, ale, too heavy meals, a sedentary life, too much studies, etc. **Nux-v.** (31)
- If it arises from rich living and is accompanied with anxious, sad dreams. **Puls.** (34)

## 157. NOSE-BLEED: See EPISTAXIS

## 158. NOSE RUNNING: See COLDS

## 159. OPHTHALMIA: See CONJUNCTIVITIS

## 160. OTITIS: See EARS, INFLAMMATION OF

## 161. OTORRHOEA *(Discharge from ears)*

- If the discharge is waxy or purulent, or if

there is much excoriation (rawness) of the
ears; or if after scarlatina. *Merc.* (30)

- If the discharge is purulent or mucous; or
if after measles or scarlatina. *Puls.* (34)

- If after scarlatina, with throbbing pain in
and about the ears. *Bell.* (9)

- For discharge from the ears, especially in
children. *Calc-p.* (12)

## 162. PAINFUL JOINTS: See JOINTS, PAINFUL

## 163. PAINS

- In case of sudden onset of severe pain after
exposure to dry cold air; great restlessness. *Acon.* (1)

- For burning, stinging, stitching pain as a
result of insect stings, or due to gout or
rheumatism, when the back feels stiff,
tired and bruised, and the symptoms are
worse from heat. *Apis* (6)

- In case of bruised sore, pains all over,
usually due to overexertion or a fall or blow,
when the bed feels too hard. *Arn.* (7)

- For violent, cutting and tearing pain in
neck, spine, or hips. *Bell.* (9)

- In case of pain in nape, back and limbs,
especially after exposure to dry cold air,
generally east wind; worse from movement. *Bry.* (11)

- In case of spasmodic chest pain due to
indigestion. *Carb-v.* (14)
*in alternation with*
*Mag-p.* (29)

- For intolerable pains which drive the
patient from bed at night to walk the floor;
arms go to sleep when grasping objects. *Cham.* (15)

- When the pains shift rapidly and spread
upwardly and are relieved by cold. *Led.* (27)

- For pains, especially in the lower part of back, which come on two hours after food, or overexertion or excessive study. **Nux-v.** (31)

- When the pains are brought on by overstraining the muscles, or exposure to cold and wet, and they are worse in cold damp weather, during rest and at night. **Rhus-t.** (35)

- For the agonising pains in abdomen, which are relieved by bending double and hard pressure and are worse on eating or drinking. **Colo.** (17) *in alternation with* **Mag-p.** (29)

- For pains before or during menses, which cause giddiness. **Mag-p.** (29)

- Especially when the pains are worse on passing urine. **Canth.** (13)

- For easily excited and emaciated (excessively lean) children, with odd pains in the hips, shins and the joints; legs weak. **Calc-p.** (12)

### 164. PANICS AND FEARS: See FEARS

### 165. PALPITATION: See HEART, PALPITATION OF

### 166. PAROTITIS: See MUMPS

### 167. PERIODS, IRREGULAR: See MENSES *(under different heads)*

### 168. PERSPIRATION *(Sweat)*

- In ease of various ailments, *viz.*, fever, croup, etc., when there is no perspiration. **Acon.** (1)
- When there is profuse perspiration on slightest movement. **Bry.** (11)
- In case of cold perspiration and cold breath. **Carb-v.** (14)

- In case of profuse, sour, sticky perspiration continuing day and night, with sensitiveness of the skin to touch. *Hep.* (23)
- When the perspiration stains the clothes yellow. *Merc.* (30)

## 169. PHOTOPHOBIA : See LIGHT INTOLERABLE

## 170. PILES *(Haemorrhoids)*

- When the disease is constitutional and is generally accompanied with irritability and constipation, intense pain, protrusion of large haemorrhoids, with itching, burning and stinging of anus, smarting pain in urination with bruised low back pain. *Nux-v.* (31)
- When much slime or mucus is discharged and the complaints are associated with indigestion, thirstlessness and easy bleeding of piles. *Puls.* (34)
- When the piles protrude like a bunch of grapes, bleed frequently, and there is much rawness, soreness and burning sensation in the anus and rectum, usually with diarrhoea and prolapsus of ani. *Aloes* (4)
- In case of profuse discharge of blood, throbbing and inflammatory symptoms. *Acon.* (1)
- When there is throbbing and bleeding with congestion of brain. *Bell.* (9)
  *in alternation with*
  *Ferr-p.* (20)
- When there is burning sensation as from hot needles and general weakness. *Ars.* (8)
- When the piles do not bleed and there is constipation and itching at anus, with fullness and throbbing headache. *Sulph.* (39)

## 171. PLEURISY

- When the inflammation, cough and fever are severe. **Acon.** (1)
- When the pains are sharp and cutting and very violent during inspiration. **Bry.** (11)

## 172. POISONING

- For poisoning, especially food poisoning, associated with severe vomiting and purging, and great weakness, restlessness coldness, chilliness and sometimes black and bloody diarrhoea. **Ars.** (8)
- If accompanied with nausea and vomiting, with colic and diarrhoea, worse on movement. **Bry.** (11)
- When associated with severe vomiting and purging, beads of cold sweat on face and forehead, and collapse. **Verat.** (40)
- In case of nausea and vomiting, with cramping pain in upper abdomen and marked collapse, icy cold body, air hunger and desire to be fanned. **Carb-v.** (14)
- Should there be fiery burning pains on passing urine and pallor of face. **Canth.** (13)
- If associated with restlessness, tossing and great fear, especially of death. **Acon.** (1)
- When due to excessive starchy or rich fatty foods, with thirstlessness. **Puls.** (34)
- When due to indigestible foods, irritability. **Nux-v.** (31)
- If accompanied with enteritis (inflammation of intestines) and colic, worse in the morning and better by hard pressure and bending double. **Colo.** (17)
in alternation with
**Mag-p.** (29)

## 173. PREGNANCY, DISORDERS OF

- In case of wind colic caused due to a chilly diarrhoea, with greenish or watery stools. **Cham.** (15)
- If the pain is very severe, and is relieved by bending double or hard pressure. **Colo.** (17)
- If the pains are of a cramping nature, or if there is much constipation. **Nux-v.** (31)
- When there are spasms in the abdomen, or if the pain is worse when sitting or lying, or when the complaints come on in the evening or at night. **Puls.** (34)
- When the complaints are as a result of mis-step, a fall, or a blow. **Arn.** (7)
- If there is debility or emaciation or excessive vomiting after eating or drinking. **Ars.** (8)

*See also* **MORNING SICKNESS**

## 174. RASH

- If there be heat, thirst and fever with restlessness. **Acon.** (1)
- If there is delirium, or if the face is bloated and the eyes are inflamed. **Bell.** (9)
- In case of lying down in women or infants, or if the rash is suppressed or undeveloped. **Bry.** (11)
- When there is great irritation, which is aggravated by warmth. **Merc.** (30)
- If the rash in attended with gastric symptoms. **Puls.** (34)

## 175. RED GUM

- If there is much fever and restlessness. **Acon.** (1)
- When the fever has abated. **Bry.** (11)

- If there is great fretfulness and excitement.  *Cham.* (15)

## 176. RESTLESSNESS

- In those with acute imagination and fearing of death predicting even the day and time of death.  *Acon.* (1)
- When accompanied with debility and exhaustion, the subject thinking his disease is incurable; he fears death, especially when alone.  *Ars.* (8)
- If with great apprehension at night.  *Rhus-t.* (35)

## 177. RHEUMATISM

- In case of high fever, or when there are violent shooting or tearing pains, aggravated by touch, with swelling of the affected parts, and high-coloured and scanty urine.  *Acon.* (1)
- When the pain is almost unbearable.  *Cham.* (15)
- In case of flying pains, worse from warmth, and better in open air and cold, especially in those with mild, yielding disposition.  *Puls.* (34)
- When the pains begin in the lower extremities and travel upward.  *Led.* (27)
- When with creeping chilliness and puffy swelling of the affected parts, worse from warmth and at night.  *Merc.* (30)
- When the parts are rigid, stiff and sore, worse during rest, cold and damp and better after continued motion and from heat.  *Rhus-t.* (35)
- When there are tearing, shooting pains, especially in joints, with shiny swelling,

- and the pains are worse on movement and better with complete rest. **Bry.** (11)
- When with a fear of being touched. **Arn.** (7)
- In case of the rheumatism of knees and low back area and large joints. **Ruta** (36)
- If there is congestion in head, with redness of the face and eyes, or if there is much swelling of the part, with widely spreading redness. **Bell.** (9)
- For rheumatism in tuberculous (scrofulous) patients and obstinate cases. **Sulph.** (39)

## 178. RINGWORM

- When there is irritation of scalp, with violent itching and small pustules at the roots of the hair. **Rhus-t.** (35)
- When the pustules dry up and the skin begins to scale off. **Sulph.** (39)

## 179. SCABIES

- For pustular (with pus) eruptions, particularly in bends of knees, with burning and itching, better from external warmth. **Ars.** (8)
- When the eruption is dry and fine, almost over the whole body, with itching, worse on extremities and undressing, with belching and passing flatus (winds). **Carb-v.** (14)
- In case of fat, pustular and crusty itch. **Hep.** (23)
- For humid supppurating eruption, full of deep fissures; itching violently when becoming warm during the day. **Lyco.** (28)
- In case of fat itch, especially in the bends of elbows, with itching all over, worse at

night when in bed (and causing sleeplessness). **Merc.** (30)

- For voluptuous tingling, itching in the bends of joints, between fingers, as soon as getting warm in bed, with burning and soreness after scratching; skin rough and scaly, with formation of little vesicles and pustules. **Sulph.** (39)

## 180. SCIATICA

- In recent cases, when the right leg is affected and the pain is very severe, paroxysmal and cramp-like which radiates down the leg to the foot, with numbness and weakness, is worse from cold and better by binding the painful part tightly. **Colo.** (17)
- In rheumatic sciatica, or if due to exposure to cold or damp, when there is a chronic condition with burning tearing pains, which are worse on beginning to move, and at rest and better from heat and continued motion. **Rhus-t** (35)
- When the pains are aggravated by motion and better from rest. **Bry.** (11)
- For sciatica in either leg, which is worse at night, from cold air, during or after sleep. **Lach.** (26)
- When the pain is intermittent, worse at night, from cold and rapid movement, and better by gentle motion and external heat. **Ars.** (8)
- When the sciatic pain is darting and shooting and the limbs are stiff, cold, weak and feel paralyzed, worse in the morning and better from heat. **Nux-v.** (31)
- If it is worse in the evening or at night, or when seated, or if arising after taking rich food. **Puls.** (34)

- In case of right-sided sciatica. **Lyco.** (28)
- For general pains, inflammation and redness of the affected parts. **Ferr-p.** (20) *in alternation with* **Mag-p.** (29)
- In case of tingling, with pain and attacks returning in cold weather, with tearing and shooting in hip-bone. **Calc-p.** (12)
- In case of prolonged suffering. **Sulph.** (39)

## 181. SEA SICKNESS: *See MOTION SICKNESS*

## 182. SHINGLES, HERPES *(A skin disease marked by development of clusters of vesicles due to viral infection)*

- In recent cases, with redness, much burning and itching in the vesicles, better from warmth and movement and worse in bed. **Rhus-t.** (35)
- When there is burning pain, restlessness, anxiety and prostration, worse after midnight and better by local heat and general warmth. **Ars.** (8)
- If there is burning, stinging pain with redness and shining and swelling, thirstlessness and restlessness. **Apis** (6)

## 183. SHOCK

- If immediately following an accident, especially if there is much fear. **Acon.** (1)
- For mental or physical shocks, recent or many years old. **Arn.** (7)

## 184. SICKNESS

- When with burning pains in abdomen. **Ars.** (8)
- Where there is constant nausea. **Ipec.** (25)

- If from over-eating and sedentary (sitting) habits. *Nux-v.* (31)
- If from rich, fat foods, with thirstlessness. *Puls.* (34)

## 185. SKIN, BURNING SENSATION OF

- For burning sensation all over the body, worse bathing, or in case of itching skin, in which scratching gives relief but results in burning and soreness; burning heat in soles and palms. *Sulph.* (39)
- In case of burning pains which are relieved by heat and covering. *Ars.* (8)
- When skin feels burning in phthisical patients. *Phos.* (32)
- For burning sensation, with restlessness and agonising tossing-about. *Acon.* (1)
- For stinging pain and burning sensation of the skin, with redness and swelling of the whole body or any part of it. *Apis.* (6)
- In case of burning sensation all over, with localized area of inflammation which feels hot, when touched. *Bell.* (9)
- When the burning sensation is felt in the abdomen, rectum or urethra. *Canth.* (13)
- For burning sensation of eyes, hands and feet, especially in bilious subjects. *Bry.* (11)

## 186. SLEEPLESSNESS *(Insomnia)*

- For sleeplessness after a shock, fright or panic, with restless tossing, or if there is associated chill, fever or rigor; sleeplessness of old age; anxious dreams. *Acon.* (1)
- When due to over-tiredness; bed feels too hard; must keep moving in search of a soft place. *Arn.* (7)

## COMMON AILMENTS AND THEIR REMEDIES

- For sleeplessness after midnight, with anxiety and restlessness; has to get up and walk on floor, or tosses around the bed. *Ars.* (8)

- In case of restless sleep with frightful dreams; jerks awake when dropping off; child tosses, starts and cries, kicks the clothes off, twitches. *Bell.* (9)

- For sleeplessness and restlessness due to pain or cramps, gets up and walks on floor; the child is irritable and wants to be carried all the time; twitching of different parts of the body. *Cham.* (15)

- When there is an overactive mind in the late evening, worrying about the day's happenings, is unable to fall asleep until the early hours, and then sleeps soundly. *Lyco.* (28)

- When due to mental strain, overwork or over-indulgence, or taking coffee or tea in excess; wakes about 2-3 a.m. and after a long wakeful period drops off and wakes late in the morning, tired and unrefreshed. *Nux-v.* (31)

- If unable to fall asleep until after midnight, then awakes again at about 3 a.m., often to walk about or have a snack or cold drink, and then falls asleep again; the patient sleeps with arms above the head, and is always worse in a warm room. *Puls.* (34)

- If due to an overactive mind in bed, or over-tiredness after a long journey, with exhaustion, irritability and slight giddiness. *Cocc.* (16)

- When there is waking or restlessness in the early hours, between 2 and 5 a.m. *Sulph.* (39)

**Note :** A luke-warm water bath or sponging the body with cold water before retiring, a well-ventilated room and complete rest to mind are of great help in getting rid of insomniac conditions.

### 187. SNEEZING: *See COLDS & CATARRHS*

## 188. SORE MOUTH: *See APHTHAE*

## 189. SOR ETHROAT

- If due to exposure to cold winds when there is dryness, roughness, burning, smarting and tingling in the throat, with high fever, and the throat is very red and painful which hurts to swallow, and the eyes are sparkling. **Acon.** (1)

- When the throat is swollen and soggy-looking, with burning, stinging pain and suffocation, and is worse in heat. **Apis** (6)

- When the throat is dry and burning, and is better by warmth. **Ars.** (8)

- When the fauces (oral cavity) and tonsils are inflamed, bright red and painful, is worse on swallowing; throat is dry, burns like fire and feels raw; the tongue is bright red and has strawberry appearance. **Bell.** (9)

- When the throat is hot and dry, speech is difficult, and the whole area is inflamed, infected and swollen; swallowing is painful, with high temperature, salivation, enlarged glands and offensive breath, yellow-coated tongue, worse at night. **Merc.** (30)

- When sore throat develops several days after exposure in warm, moist weather; difficult swallowing. **Gels.** (21)

- When the throat is very irritable, with a sense of fish-bone stuck in it, and is worse from cold or draught. **Hep.** (23)

- When the complaints begin in the left side of the throat and tend to travel towards right; the throat is bluish in colour and is worse on swallowing liquids; intolerant of any pressure in the neck area; better for solid food. **Lach.** (26)

- When the complaints begin in the right side of the throat and tend to travel towards the left. **Lyco. (28)**
- In case of disordered stomach, usually in persons of sedentary (sitting) habits or due to swotting (over-study). **Nux-v. (31)**
- For inflammation and burning pains, redness and dryness of throat, with hoarseness and loss of voice. **Ferr-p. (20)**
- If the glands under the jaws are swollen, or if it arises from the slightest chill, with hoarseness and tickling in the trachea (windpipe). **Cham. (15)**
- In case of enlarged tonsils, sorethroat, with aching and pain on swallowing. **Calc-p. (12)**

## 189. SPLINTERS, SENSATION OF

- For any deep, circumscribed (bounded) wounds, with infection, redness and local formation of pus. **Led. (27)**
- When there is a sensation of splinter(s) at the back of the throat. **Hep. (23)**

## 190. SPRAINS, STRAINS

- In case of sprains or strains due to overwork; sprain around a joint, with swelling and pain, bleeding in tissues. **Arn. (7)**
- When the sprain is due to fall or injury, and there is stiffness and swelling of the parts with pain, which is worse on beginning to move, from cold or damp or at rest, and better by continued motion and stretching the limbs. **Rhus-t. (35)**
- When there is severe bruising due to sprains of ankles and feet, and the sprained

- parts are cold to touch, but better with cold applications. **Led.** (27)
- If from strain of flexor (muscles that flex) tendons, usually due to sprains and injury to ligaments, when the pain is worse for stretching the limbs. **Ruta** (36)
- If the joints are involved and there is swelling, with pain which is aggravated by motion. **Bry.** (11)

## 191. STIFF NECK

- When brought on by exposure to dry cold winds, accompanied with restlessness and anxiety, and tearing in the nape of neck, with pain. **Acon.** (1)
- For painful stiff neck, worse for touch and motion. **Bry.** (11)
- When due to sudden jerk or over-straining the neck muscles, and the pain travels down back. **Rhus-t.** (35)

## 192. STINGS AND BITES: *See STINGS*

## 193. STOMACH UPSETS

- In case of gastritis (inflammation of stomach) caused by cold drinks or getting chilled. **Acon.** (1)
- When the trouble, especially gastritis, is caused by ice-creams, or when there is burning or burning pain in the stomach. **Ars.** (8)
- For acidity of stomach, with empty eructations. **Carb-v.** (14)
- In case of bitter stomach and water-brash (eructation of acid or gastric contents from stomach into mouth). **Bry.** (11)

- For disorders brought on by fats and oily foods, with thirstlessness. **Puls.** (34)
- In case of belching and flatulence, worse from 4 p.m. to 8 p.m. **Lyco.** (28)

## 194. STOMATITIS: See APHTHAE

## 195. STRAINS: See SPRAINS

## 196. STYES: See EYELIDS, INFLAMMATION OF

## 197. SUNBURN

- When with redness, heat and throbbing; sun-stroke (convulsion, coma and high fever from exposure to sun). **Bell.** (9)
- When a reaction is expected after remaining in the sun for a day. **Canth.** (13)

## 198. SUNSTROKE *(High fever, convulsion, coma from excessive exposure to sun)*

- In case of red, hot, flushed face, with violent headache, bounding full pulse, dilated pupils, blood-shot eyes, severe throbbing of carotids, worse for jar or noise and usually associated with violent dizziness, delirium, or sudden falling-down, as if from apoplexy. **Bell.** (9)
- In case of waves of terrible, bursting, pulsating headache, which is worse from motion and jar, with pale face, fixed eyes, vomiting, bounding pulse and heavy breathing, with sudden upward rush of blood to head, as if it would burst. **Glon.** (22)
- In case of feverishness and right-sided headache, accompanied with irritability and dizziness. **Gels.** (21)

- When the inflammatory and respiratory symptoms are present. *Ferr-p.* (20)

**Note :** Immediately loosen the clothes and remove the victim in a shade or dark room. Give plenty of cold drinks and sponge the body with tepid water at frequent intervals.

## 199. SWEATS: *See PERSPIRATION*

## 200. SYNCOPE: *See FAINTING*

## 201. TEETHING: *See DENTITION*

## 202. THIRST

- In case of complete loss of thirst, usually in those who are always worse for heat and suffer from puffy swellings. *Apis* (6)
- When the patient is totally thirstless even though the mouth may be dry. *Puls.* (34)
- In case of excessive thirst with high temperature and great restlessness. *Acon.* (1)
- If there is great thirst at longer intervals and the patient drinks plenty of cold water at a time. *Bry.* (11)
- When with dry mouth and thirst, and a desire for milk. *Rhus-t.* (35)
- Thirstlessness with fever. *Gels.* (21)

## 203. THROAT RELAXED

- If the uvula (fleshy body suspended from palate) or the soft palate (roof of mouth) is inflamed, or swollen, or if the relaxation arises from derangement of the digestive organs. *Nux-v.* (31)

## 204. THROAT, SORE: See SORE THROAT

## 205. TONSILLITIS *(Inflammation of tonsils)*

- When there is a tendency for tonsillitis after riding in cold winds. **Acon.** (1)
- When the tonsil, especially right-sided, is bright red, swollen and acutely painful, and is worse on swallowing; the neck is often stiff and inflamed. **Bell.** (9)
- If the tonsils are swollen and raw, with great pain on swallowing, and fever. **Ferr-p.** (20)
- In case of chronic tonsillitis, with purulent infection and sensation like splinter or fish-bone in the throat, when swallowing. **Hep.** (23)
- When the left-sided tonsil is involved and the patient finds it difficult to swallow liquids; the tonsil is blue and swollen. **Lach.** (26)
- In case the right-sided tonsil is affected. **Lyco.** (28)
- When the tonsils and fauces are dry, acutely painful and yellowish-red, often covered with a thin false membrane (sheet) and the tongue is flabby with imprints of teeth; the pain is usually worse by swallowing or speech. **Merc.** (30)
- In case of red inflammatory swelling of throat with sticking or stinging pain on tonsils. **Rhus-t.** (35)
- When the tonsils are large, pale and inflamed; hearing may be impaired. **Calc-p.** (12)

## 206. TOOTHACHE

- For toothache in nervous and fearful subjects, if there is much feverishness, or the patient is beside himself with trauma, or the pains are one-sided, but are difficult

- to describe, and are aggravated by cold wind and better for cold water. ***Acon.*** (1)
- In case of toothache after filling or after tooth extraction. ***Arn.*** (7)
- In case of severe, intolerable pain, driving the patient almost to despair, with heat and swelling of the cheek, or if the pain affects one whole side of the head, with irritability, and when the pain is worse at night, in a warm room or in cold air, by taking anything warm and drinking coffee. ***Cham.*** (15)
- In case of neuralgic nervous type of pain, relieved by heat and hot fluids. ***Mag-p.*** (29)
- When there is stabbing, throbbing pain in the gums, with dry mouth, much heat and congestion about the head. ***Bell.*** (9)
- When the teeth are painful and feel too long, and are sensitive to touch, and are worse in cold air. ***Plant.*** (33)
- In case of decayed teeth, with tearing shooting pains, swelling of cheeks, gums or glands, much salivation, pain in the whole side of the head, or extending to the ears and head and the pain is worse during night, from both hot and cold, and better by rubbing the cheeks. ***Merc.*** (30)
- In case of throbbing or dragging and shifting pains, extending from the decayed tooth to the eye, worse from warm things, in a warm room, in the evening and in bed, and better by cold air and water. ***Puls.*** (34)
- For rheumatic toothache, worse in warmth and better by cold applications. ***Bry.*** (11)
- For toothache from stimulants or coffee, with indigestion and irregular action of bowels, when the pain is worse at night, in

the morning on waking, or when engaged
in mental work. ***Nux-v.*** (31)

- In case of inflammatory toothache, with soreness, bleeding after tooth extraction. ***Ferr-p.*** (20)
- For toothache and other digestive disturbances during dentition. ***Calc-p.*** (12)

**Note :** Put a cotton plug soaked with *Plantago* φ on the affected tooth to have instant relief from pain.

## 207. TRAVEL SICKNESS: *See MOTION SICKNESS*

## 208. URINARY DISORDERS

- In case of acute inflammation of urinary organs, with frequent urination, burning pain and discomfort before, during and after urination, which sometimes is very painful and passes in drops. ***Canth.*** (13)
- When the urine is retained due to a relaxed or paralytic condition of the neck of the bladder. ***Gels.*** (21)
- If the condition follows an abuse of foods, wine or other spirituous liquors, when the urine is retained with great difficulty and passes involuntarily, or when there are burning tearing pains, with ineffectual urging to urinate, with an acute feeling of a full bladder, with spasmodic closure of urethra. ***Nux-v.*** (31)
- For retention of urine from a blow or fall, or other mechanical injuries or from the irritation of calculi (stone). ***Arn.*** (7).
- In case of incontinence of urine from cold or syphilis. ***Merc.*** (30)
- When incontinence (unable to restrain) of

- urine is due to muscular weakness. **Ferr-p.** (20)
- In case of constant urging to urinate, when standing or walking, and for spasmodic retention of urine. **Mag-p.** (29)
- For enuresis (involuntary urine) in old people, with frequent urging to urinate. **Calc-p.** (12)

## 209. URTICARIA *(Nettle-rash)*

- In case of severe acute allergic cases when there is much fever, great restlessness, agitation, anxiety and collapse. **Acon.** (1)
- When caused due to eating fish, or by damp weather, with burning and stinging, and the symptoms are worse in bed or during rest and better with continued motion. **Rhus-t.** (35)
- If it chiefly affects the joints, or arises from damp weather, or if the eruption disappears suddenly and is followed by difficulty of breathing; or if there are chest symptoms. **Bry.** (11)
- If there is feverishness. **Ferr-p.** (20)
- If the head becomes affected and there is delirium, with sore throat. **Bell.** (9)
- When the eruptions are swollen and are accompanied with stinging, burning and itching, relieved by cold applications. **Apis** (6)
- If accompanied with itching, swelling and much burning, relieved by local heat and warmth, in general. **Ars.** (8)
- If caused due to indigestion, or gastric derangements, or dysmenorrhoea (painful menses), or after taking rich, fatty food, pastries, etc. **Puls.** (34)

- In chronic cases, with swelling, itching and redness, worse on bathing. **Sulph.** (39)

## 210. VARICOSE (DILATED) VEINS

- When due to fatigue and long periods of standing. **Acon.** (1)
- When following childbirth. **Puls.** (34)
- When there is associated poor circulation. **Carb-v.** (14)

## 211. VERTIGO, GIDDINESS, DIZZINESS

- For vertigo, with a feeling as if intoxicated upon rising, or by motion of a carriage or vessel. **Cocc.** (16)
- When the vertigo seems to spread from occiput (back part of the head), with blurred vision. **Gels.** (21)
- In case of vertigo on rising from a seat, with biliousness (excessive secretion of bile) and tendency to pitch forward. **Bry.** (11)
- In case of giddiness arising from stomach, with constipation, in persons of spare habits, or if during or after meals or when walking in the open air, or with fainting, whirling of the head and danger of falling down. **Nux-v.** (31)
- For giddiness from rush of blood to head, with flushing, throbbing or pressing pain. **Ferr-p.** (20)
- If the vertigo or giddiness is felt on raising the head, when lying or stooping and there is much redness of face. **Acon.** (1)
- For vertigo from optical defects, with dark spots floating before the eyes. **Mag-p.** (29)
- When with vertigo, there is partial loss of consciousness, staggering, or fullness and violent pressure in the forehead. **Bell.** (9)

- If the vertigo arises from eating fatty or rich foods, like pastries, etc., or if there is relief in the open air, or if it is accompanied with nausea or with feeling, as though intoxicated.                                          *Puls.* (34)

## 212. VOMITING

- If from nervous upset or fright.                  *Acon.* (1)
- In case of vomiting with severe cutting abdominal pains, better by bending double and hard pressure.                          *Colo.* (17)
- If from over-loading the stomach, or taking rich, fatty foods; without thirst.        *Puls.* (34)
- If there is simple nausea or vomiting after eating and drinking, or if accompanied with diarrhoea and vomiting.            *Ipec.* (25)
- In case of constant vomiting and purging, with cold sweat on forehead, great thirst, prostration, and coldness of entremities  *Verat.* (40)
- In case of nausea and vomiting from riding a carriage, boat, train or car, or due to loss of sleep at night.                     *Cocc.* (16)
- When the child is intolerant of milk and vomits it in large curds as soon as taken.  *Aeth.* (2)
- If from biliousness or from weakness of stomach, or after drinking wines or spirits, worse in early morning.               *Nux-v.* (31)
- If there is violent vomiting of everything taken or attending diarrhoea and burning in stomach, great prostration and thirst for frequent sips of water.                      *Ars.* (8)
- In case of vomiting of cold drinks as soon as they become warm in the stomach.    *Phos.* (32)

COMMON AILMENTS AND THEIR REMEDIES 115

### 213. WATERBRASH: *See ACIDITY and HEARTBURN*

### 214. WHITES: *See LEUCORRHOEA*

### 215. WHOOPING COUGH

- If there is a hard dry cough, which is worse at night, or if there be headache, or sore-throat, or symptoms of congestion in the head. *Bell.* (9)
- If from very beginning, the cough is attended with suffocative symptoms, and bluish face. *Ipec.* (25)
- If there is a dry fatiguing cough attended with vomiting, danger of suffocation and bluish face. *Nux-v.* (31)
- If from commencement the cough is loose, with vomiting of mucus or food, or is attended with a mucous diarrhoea. *Puls.* (34)
- If the violence of paroxysms remains unabated, or if there be great weakness, or suffocative fits. *Verat.* (40)

### 216. WORMS

- If there are feverish symptoms at night with restlessness and great debility. *Acon.* (1)
- In case of worm-diarrhoea or colic, distension of the bowels, straining at stool, with small slimy evacuation or bleeding from the nose, cause by worms. *Merc.* (30)

### 217. WOUND, CUTS, INJURIES

- For injuries to soft parts from blow or fall, or concussion of brain, or if there is shock. *Arn* (7)
- For injuries to parts rich in nerves and tail

- bone (coccyx); extreme sensitiveness of punctured wounds; spinal concussion; violent pain. **Hyper** (24) *to be alternated with* **Arn.** (7)

- For injuries to eye, the eyeball turning black. **Led.** (27) *to be alternated with* **Arn.** (7)

- For punctured wounds which feel cold to touch; also for injuries to eye when the eyeball turns black. **Led.** (27) *to be alternated with* **Hyper.** (24)

- If after an injury to head, pain persists in the back part with great heaviness of eyelids and tremulousness (shaking) of limbs. **Gels.** (21)

- When the punctured wounds become red and are very sensitive to touch, with burning, stinging pains. **Apis** (6)

- For sprains, bruises, cuts, wounds, etc., with pain and congestion. **Ferr-p.** (20)

- If the cut or wound is infected and suppurates (gets pus). **Hep.** (23)

- If the cut or wound is painful and hot. **Acon.** (1)

- In case the cut or wound is painful, red and swollen, with high temperature and headache. **Bell.** (9)

**Note:** In case of abrasions, scratches and superficial wounds, apply *Calendula lotion* externally (10 drops of *Calendula* φ to be mixed in 40 drops of boiled cool water along with the internal administration of the indicated remedies).

## 218. YELLOWNESS OF SKIN

- If accompanied with the signs and symptoms of jaundice. **Bry.** (11)
- When due to anaemia. **Ferr-p.** (20) *in alternation with* **Calc-p.** (12)

# 11 | THE LEADING CHARACTERISTICS OF THE RECOMMENDED REMEDIES

## 1. ACONITE NAPELLUS
### (Acon.)

1. Aphonia (loss of voice), tonsillitis, croup, laryngitis, bronchitis, pneumonia, pleurisy, otitis (inflammation of ear) and other inflammatory diseases from exposure to cold winds.
2. Retention of urine from shock.
3. Amenorrhoea in plethoric (full-blooded) young girls after fright.
4. Complaints after hair-cut.
5. Pains are unbearable, they drive him to despair or make him crazy; worse at night, make him toss about in agony; facial neuralgia (nerve pain), toothache, orchitis (inflammation of testicles), pleurisy, pericarditis (inflammation of the membrane covering heart), etc.
6. Asthma from active hyperaemia (excess of blood) of lungs.
7. *Fever:* Skin dry hot; face red, or pale and red alternately; burning thirst for large quantities of cold water; with intense, nervous restlessness, anxiety and fear; whole body burning hot.
8. Convulsions of teething children with high fever.
9. *Haemorrhages*: Bright red blood; with anxiety and fear of death.
10. *Dysentery*: When *Merc.*, though indicated, fails.

11. Incarcerated (occluded) hernia with vomiting of bile great anxiety and fear of death.
12. *Ailments:* From intense cold of winter or extreme heat of sun; suppressed perspiration; excitement; shock; anger; fright; excessive joy.
13. *Ailments*: With vanishing of sight suddenly; fainting; red face becomes pale on rising from recumbent position; hot dry skin; unconquerable anxiety, restlessness; anxiety with fear, fear of death; predicts the time of death.
14. Sciatica attended with or succeeded by numbness of the affected parts.
15. Ailments from bad effects of fear still remaining.
16. **Especially adapted to those:**
    (a) who are fearful; afraid to go out into a crowd or where there is any excitement or many people; to cross the street; great fear and anxiety in mind with ailments; life is rendered miserable by fear; is sure his disease will prove fatal; predicts the day and time of his death;
    (b) who are anxious, restless, do everything in great haste; must change position often; everything startles them; remain disquiet;
    (c) to whom music is unbearable, makes them sad;
    (d) who are disposed to mental, nervous troubles, congestions, haemorrhages, neuralgias (nerve pain).

## 2. AETHUJA CYNAPIUM
### (Aethuja)

1. Intolerance of milk; cannot bear milk in any form; it is vomited in large curds as soon as taken.
2. Complete absence of thirst.
3. Great weakness; unable to hold up the head.
4. Indigestion of teething children; violent sudden vomiting of a frothy, milk-white substance; or yellow fluid followed by curdled milk and cheesy matter.

THE LEADING CHARACTERISTICS OF THE RECOMMENDED REMEDIES  119

5. Prostration and sleepiness immediately after vomiting or diarrhoea.

6. Cramps and convulsions with clenched thumbs, red face, eyes turned downwards, pupils fixed and dilated; foam at mouth; jaws locked; pulse small, hard and quick.

7. Features expressive of pain and anxiety.

8. Idiocy in children; confused; incapacity to think.

## 3. ALLIUM CEPA
(All.-c.)

1. Colds, flu and acute sinusitis; profuse watery and acrid nasal discharge with profuse bland lachrymation (watering), worse in a warm room and better in open air.

2. Acrid, watery discharge dropping from tip of nose, burns and corrodes the nose and upper lip.

3. Burning, biting and smarting in the eyes as from smoke, must rub them; eyes watery and suffused.

4. Violent sneezing on rising from bed.

5. Catarrhal (discharging) laryngitis; cough compels patient to grasp the larynx; feels as if cough would tear it.

6. Neuralgic (nerve) pains like a long thread: in face, head, neck, chest.

7. Sore and raw spots on feet, especially heels, from friction, as of shoes.

8. **Especially adapted to:**

   (a) indolent, "weary" persons, averse to either mental or physical labour; mental labour fatigues;

   (b) old people, generally women of relaxed, phlegmatic (cold, sluggish and apathetic) habits; extreme prostration, with perspiration.

## 4. ALOE SOCOTRINA
### (Aloes)

1. *Diarrhoea*: Sudden, imperative; with much flatulence; early morning, driving the patient out of bed; after beer; after oysters; involuntary; unreliable sphincter of anus, with jelly-like stools; alternates with headache; rumbling before stool.
2. *Constipation:* Stool has to be removed mechanically; causes headache, passes hard stool involuntarily.
3. *Haemorrhoids:* Blue, like bunch of grapes; better from cold water or cold applications; with prolapse of rectum.
4. Itches appear each year, as winter approaches.
5. Itching and burning in anus preventing sleep.
6. Diseases of mucous membranes, causing the production of mucus in jelly-like lumps from throat or rectum.

## 5. ANTIMONIUM TARTARICUM
### (Ant-t.)

1. Vertigo alternates with drowsiness.
2. Broncho-pneumonia or respiratory diseases with flapping of nostrils.
3. Ailments from bad effects of vaccination.
4. Asphyxia neonatorum (imperfect breathing in the new-born).
5. Foreign bodies in trachea or larynx.
6. Jaundice with pneumonia.
7. Resolution stage of pneumonia with rattling in chest.
8. Acute chest complaints of children with pale and sickly face, covered with cold sweat; the eyes are sunken; nostrils are dilated and flapping; rattling of phlegm in the chest; child is in a comatose condition.

9. Catarrhal (mucus discharging) disease in broken-down old persons, having lack of reaction; worse in cold damp weather; white expectoration with dyspnoea, must sit up.
10. Gouty complaints, worse in cold damp weather; gouty arthritis.
11. Gonorrhoeal ophthalmia (inflammation of the eye).
12. Rheumatic pains in the teeth with rheumatic pains in the joints.
13. Gastric complaints with loathing of food, nausea and vomiting; inability to digest; with thirstlessness; desire for acids and sour fruits; aversion to milk.
14. Bleeding ulcers in the stomach with other characteristic symptoms of the remedy.
15. Dropsy of lower extremities with gastric or catarrhal symptoms.
16. Chicken-pox, small-pox; pus-filled eruptions leaving a bluish red mark.
17. **Especially suited to the following types of patients:**
    (a) who have great sleepiness or irresistible inclination to sleep with nearly all complaints;
    (b) children who want to be carried during their illnesses;
    (c) children who will not let you feel the pulse; cry and whine, if any one touches them; want to be left alone when sick; peevish;
    (d) who have hydrogenoid (moisture-affecting) constitution; are susceptible to damp cold weather;
    (e) who desire apples, fruits and acids generally;
    (f) infants and children allergic to milk, vomit it immediately.

## 6. APIS MELLIFICA
### (Apis)

1. Ailments from jealousy, fright, rage, vexation, bad news, mental shock.

2. Bad effects of acute exanthema (eruptions) imperfectly developed or suppressed; measles, scarlatina, urticaria. suppressed eruptions.
3. *Oedema* (puffiness): Pitting on pressure; marked under the eyes; of hands and feet; dropsy without thirst.
4. *Pain*: Burning, stinging, sore; suddenly migrating from one part to other.
5. *Diarrhoea*: In eruptive diseases, especially if eruption be suppressed; of drunkards; involuntary from every motion; with anus wide open (*Phos.*).
6. Albuminuria (albumin in urine) after scarlatina when *Canth.* has failed.
7. Meningitis with sudden shrill, piercing screams, rolling of head from side to side; opisthotonos (arching backward), or head drawn back, gnashing of teeth.
8. Chemosis (swelling) of conjunctiva with sharp pains.
9. *Right-sided troubles*: Right-sided ovarian cyst, hydrocele.
10. Synovitis (inflammation of membrane containing joint fluids), with burning, sore, stinging pains; worse from warm applications.
11. Sore throat with constrictive sensation.
12. *Intermittent fevers:* Chill at 3 p.m.; chill with thirst; feels worse in a warm room.
13. Menstrual troubles in women with burning, stinging pains and thirstlessness with great heat.
14. Scirrhus or open cancer with enlarged, indurated glands with characteristic and constitutional symptoms of *Apis*.
15. **Especially suited to the following types of patients:**
    (a) who are warm-blooded; worse in warm and closed room;
    (b) children, girls and women, though generally careful, become awkward and let things fall, while handling them;
    (c) irritable, nervous, fidgety persons hard to please;
    (d) who have a weeping disposition; cannot help crying; discouraged and despondent;

(e) who are extremely sensitive to touch (*Bell., Hep., Lach.*);
(f) who are worse after sleeping, touch and pressure, heat of bed and at 3 p.m. and better from sitting erect, changing position, walking, uncovering and bathing;
(g) jealous persons; women, especially widows;
(h) persons who are apathetic, are absent-minded, cannot concentrate; are listless, fault-finding, joyless, suspicious or indolent;
(i) sad and melancholic;
(j) foolish persons.

# 7. ARNICA MONTANA
## (Arn.)

1. Bad effects of mechanical injuries even of remote origin.
2. Bruised pain, soreness, haemorrhage, extravasation (escape into tissues) of blood, epistaxis (nose-bleed) after a fall or blow from a blunt weapon.
3. Concussion with stupor, meningitis, shock after head-injury.
4. Black eye, retinal haemorrhage from a blow to the eye; or severe cough.
5. *Apoplexy* (stroke): Helps in the absorption of blood.
6. *Paralysis:* Left-sided with full and strong pulse; sighing, muttering and stertorous breathing; with unconsciousness.
7. *Gout of great toe:* With great fear of being touched or struck by a person coming near him.
8. Prevents post-delivery haemorrhage and other complications, if given just after delivery.
9. Hypertrophy (enlargement) of heart from heart strain and over-work.
10. Retention of urine from injuries or constant dribbling of urine after labour.

11. **Especially adapted to:**
    (a) sanguine, plethoric (full-blooded) persons of very red face and lively expression;
    (b) nervous persons who cannot bear pain;
    (c) persons who remain long impressed by even slightest mechanical injuries;
    (d) apathetic persons who say, "There is nothing the matter with him," even when they are seriously ill, send the doctor away and want to be left alone;
    (e) patients who worry and exaggerate trivial symptoms;
    (f) patients who are sullen, morose, do not speak a word, do not want to be talked to;
    (g) patients who are fearful but fear remains at night after an accident;
    (h) horror of instant death with cardiac distress at night.

## 8. ARSENICUM ALBUM
### (Ars.)

1. *Ailments from:* Alcohol, chewing tobacco, sausage-poisoning, dissecting wounds, bites of venomous insects, anthrax (carbuncle), sea-bathing, ptomaine poisoning, malaria, abuse of quinine, iodine, climbing mountains.
2. Ailments from care, worry, grief, fright and shock.
3. Ailments with great prostration and rapid sinking of vital force, rapid emaciation, despair of recovery; worse when alone; aggravated from physical exertion.
4. Burning pains relieved from warm applications.
5. Vomiting and diarrhoea with anxiety and restlessness after taking ice-cream.
6. *Cholera:* With cold perspiration, thirst for small quantities of water, extreme prostration, cadaveric appearance, foul stools and vomits, restlessness, anxiety and fear of ath.
7. *Dropsy* (puffiness): With thirst for small quantities of water, restlessness, anxiety and prostration.

# THE LEADING CHARACTERISTICS OF THE RECOMMENDED REMEDIES

8. *Anaemia:* Cancerous affections; collapse; fainting; inflammations; gangrene; ulcers; psoriasis; scabies; urticaria; coryza; hay fever; aphthae (whitish spots in mouth); fissured tongue; diphtheria; dysentery; diabetes; leucorrhoea; asthma; pneumonia; pericarditis (inflammation of heart covering); phthisis; syphilis.
9. *Delirium:* With depression, restlessness, fear of death, fear of being alone; suicidal tendency.
10. Acute nephritis following exanthemata (eruptive disease), with convulsions; puffiness of face, mental anguish and suppressed urine; with uraemic delusions (*Canth.*)
11. *Herpes Zoster:* Pains burning, shooting, sticking; worse at night; with restlessness, thirst for small quantities of water, black colour of the exudate.
12. *Anaemia:* After acute fevers, haemorrhages, with inability to retain food or drink due to irritability of stomach; great restlessness.
13. **Especially suitable for persons:**
    (a) who are extremely fastidious, critical and tidy;
    (b) who are chilly, worse from cold, cold drinks, cold food, better from heat and covering;
    (c) who are anxious, restless, fearful, depressed and melancholic;
    (d) who are vexed easily, irritable, peevish and full of anguish;
    (e) who are allergic to ice-cream, fruits, bad meat, fish, strong cheese;
    (f) teething children are pale, weak, fretful, want to be carried rapidly;
    (g) who are worse after midnight (1 to 2 a.m.);
    (h) who cannot bear the smell or sight of food.

## 9. BELLADONNA
### (Bell.)

1. Ailments with rush of blood to head and face.
2. *Violent Delirium:* Disposition to bite, spit, strike and tear things; breaks into fits of laughter and gnashes the teeth;

wants to bite and strike the attendants; tries to escape.
3. *Hallucinations:* Sees ghosts, hideous faces and various insects; black animals, dogs, wolves; fears imaginary things, wants to run away from them. Delusions horrible. Convulsions come on suddenly; with high fever; during teething; with hot head and cold feet.
4. *Pains:* Come suddenly, last indefinitely and cease suddenly; renal colic.
5. *Headache:* Congestive, with red face, throbbing of brain and carotids (neck arteries), worse from slight noise, jar, motion, light, lying down, least exertion; better from pressure, tight bandaging (*Arg. Nit.*), wrapping up, during menses.
6. *Vertigo:* When stooping; when rising after stooping; on every change of position (*Bry.*).
7. Tonsillitis after riding in a cold wind.
8. *Appendicitis:* Pain in right ileo-caecal (right lower half of abdomen) region; aggravated by slightest touch, even of the bed-cover.
9. *Scarlet Fever:* Rash of a uniform, smooth, shining, scarlet redness.
10. **Prolapse of Uterus:** Sensation as if the contents of abdomen would issue through the vulva; better from standing and sitting erect; worse from lying down.
11. **Especially adapted to the persons:**
    (a) who are lively and entertaining when well, but violent and often delirious when sick;
    (b) who are plethoric, vigorous and intellectual;
    (c) *chilly persons:* great proneness to take cold; sensitive to draught of air, especially when uncovering the head;
    (d) who have reactive excitability; reaction to medicine is so quick and so sudden that they at once feel relieved;
    (e) who are hypersensitive to touch, motion, jar, light and noise, extremes of heat and cold; they are worse from lying down, at night, after midnight, after 3 p.m., looking at bright, shining objects, uncovering the head;

(f) who feel better by rest, standing or sitting erect; in a warm room;

(g) who are of tuberculous disposition.

## 10. BORAX
### (Bor.)

1. Aphthous stomatitis (ulcers in mouth); white patches with red areolae; during dentition, hot mouth, hot urine, making the child cry, when urinating.

2. *Entropion:* Eye-lashes turn inward, causing inflammation of eyes, especially at the outer canthus, where the margin of lids are very sore.

3. *Blepharitis* (Inflammation of eyelids): With margins of lids very sore; agglutination (sticking) of lids after sleep.

4. *Leucorrhoea:* Profuse, albuminous, starchy, with sensation as if warm water were flowing down; for two weeks between menses, acrid; like the white of an egg.

5. Sore mouth from plates of teeth; aggravation after eating salty or sour food.

6. Slightest injuries suppurate (form pus).

7. **Especially adapted to persons:**

    (a) who have fear and anxiety from downward motion: going downstairs, descending in the aeroplane, down the hill;

    (b) children awake suddenly, screaming and grasping sides of cradle, without apparent cause, as if frightened by a dream;

    (c) excessively nervous persons, easily frightened by the slightest noise or an unusual sharp sound, a cough, sneeze, a cry, lighting a match, etc.;

    (d) persons allergic to smoking which may bring on diarrhoea;

    (e) young women with shining red nose.

## 11. BRYONIA ALBA
### (Bry.)

1. *Ailments from:* Chagrin, anger, mortification, fright, chilling when overheated; exposure to cold; when warm weather sets in after cold days; cold drinks or ice in hot weather; suppressed discharges; menses; rash of acute exanthema (eruption), after eating beans, peas, cabbage, bread, flatulent food, fruits.

2. Complaints are worse from slightest motion, exertion, jar, swallowing, coughing, sneezing, ascending, motion of ship, lying on painless side, rising from lying, stooping, motion of eyes.

3. *Complaints are better from* lying on painful side, when quiet, during rest, pressure, dark room, cool open air, cold water, cold food.

4. *Ailments are attended with* dryness of mucous membranes with thirst for large quantities of water; constant motion of left arm and left leg; pressure as from stone at pit of stomach, relieved (through another outlet) by eructation; delirium, talks constantly about his business; desires to get out of bed and go home; vicarious menstruation: nose-bleed when menses should appear; vertigo on stooping; throbbing in head; tongue coated thick, whitish-yellow; nausea and vomiting; urine dark and scanty; high fever with profuse sweat which ameliorates.

5. *Acute meningitis* from suppressed rash of exanthematous (eruptive) fevers with constant chewing motion of mouth; face congested, puffy; temperature high, copious sweats; dry lips, thirst for large quantities of water; quiet; uncovers the body.

6. *Delirium* in acute infectious fevers, talks constantly about his business; desires to get out of bed and go home; constant motion of left arm and leg.

7. *Headache* : In morning after rising or on first opening eyes; commencing in the morning, gradually increasing until evening; from ironing, with constipation, on cough-

ing, when stooping as if brain would burst through forehead.

8. *Pains* : Stitching, tearing; worse by motion, inspiration, coughing, at night; better from absolute rest and lying on painful side.

9. *Acute Pleurisy:* When the fever has somewhat abated; pains are stitching or tearing, worse from coughing, movement, sneezing, even breathing is painful. It comes in after *Aconite*. Friction-rub present.

10. Acute inflammation of mammae (breasts) —hot and painful, heavy, stonishly hard; must support the breasts; pain worse from slightest motion.

11. *Cough :* Dry, spasmodic; with gagging and vomiting; with stitches inside of chest; with headache, worse after eating, drinking, entering a warm room, a deep inspiration.

12. *Constipation :* No inclination from inactive rectum; stools large, hard, dark, dry, as if burnt; on going to sea.

13. *Diarrhoea :* During a spell of hot weather; bilious, acrid with soreness of anus; like dirty water; of undigested food; from cold drinks when overheated; from fruits, worse in morning or moving even a hand or foot.

14. *Diabetes:* Dryness of lips and mouth, thirst for large quantities of water, persistent bitter taste in mouth; from warmth and exertion; beans, peas, cabbage, bread, fruits and flatulent (gas forming) food disagree.

15. *Acute Hepatitis* (Inflammation of liver): Liver is congested, inflamed and enlarged; stitching pains in the right hypochondrium (sides of upper abdomen), worse from motion or changing position; better from lying on the right or painful side; jaundice brought on by a fit of anger.

16. *Acute Pericarditis* (Inflammation of membrane covering heart): Of rheumatic origin, stitching pains worse from movement; better from lying on painful side; friction-rub is present.

17. *Pneumonia :* It comes after *Acon.* and *Ferr-p.* The patient is not restless; cough is moist, sharp stitching pleuritic pains, worse from coughing and any movement; tongue

**BRYONIA ALBA**            **BRYONIA ALBA**

dry and coated, thirst excessive; with delirium or constipation.

18. *Acute Rheumatism* : Joints red, hot and swollen; painful on slightest motion; touch and pressure aggravate; pains stitching or tearing in character, copious exudation in joints, with perspiration which relieves suffering.

19. *Typhoid fever* : Develops sluggishly; with headache, dry mouth, tongue coated, thirst for large quantities of water; lies quietly, with delirium, constipation, soreness of body; likes cool open air; worse in warm and closed room.

20. *Tuberculosis:* Dry teasing cough as if the head and chest would burst; sharp stitching pains in the sides; inability to take a deep breath on account of aggravation of pains.

21. **Especially adapted to the following types of patients:**

    (a) children who dislike to be carried or to be raised; fretful;

    (b) children who desire things immediately which are not to be had, or which when offered are refused; peevish;

    (c) patients who are irritable, inclined to be vehement and angry; nervous;

    (d) who have black hair, dark complexion, firm muscular fibres; dry, slender people;

    (e) who are worse from slightest motion and better from rest; although restless, wants to keep quiet and still;

    (f) who are anxious, angered easily and are obstinate;

    (g) who are warm-blooded: worse from warmth, summer; better from cool open air, cold water, cold food;

    (h) who are plethoric and venous (full-blooded) in their make-up; face is puffed and purplish;

    (i) who are of a sluggish nature; complaints develop slowly;

    (j) who are fearful: fear of death, fear of poverty.

## 12. CALCAREA PHOSPHORICA
### (Calc-p.)

1. **Especially adapted to:**
   (a) persons, especially children, who are thin, emaciated in neck, have sunken abdomen; rickety, late closure of skull bones, late in standing and walking; suffer from dentitional diarrhoea and deformed bones;
   (b) girls at puberty, tall, growing rapidly, tendency of bones to soften or spinal curvature;
   (c) persons with tendency to emaciate, albuminuria, phosphaturia (albumin and phosphate in urine), anaemia, polypi, spermatorrhoea (involuntary excessive loss of semen), scrofula (tuberculous glands) and non-union of fractured bones.

2. It is a specific remedy for hydrocephalus (increase of cerebral fluid), Bright's disease (kidney disease with albumin in urine), chorea, consumption, fistula, rheumatism, rickets, spina bifida (cleft of the spine with meningeal protrusion) and enlarged tonsils, when its characteristic symptoms are present.

**Note:** Large doses are useless and injurious. Prolonged administration has produced nephritic colic and caused passage of small calculi (stones). Low potencies are contra-indicated in old people.

## 13. CANTHARIS
### (Canth.)

1. In burns before blisters form and when they have formed, for the burning sensation. External applications give relief immediately.
2. Renal calculi (stones) with passing of urine, drop by drop, with burning sensation; constant pulling of the penis.
3. First stage of gonorrhoea with constant urging to urinate, passing a few drops at a time with blood and intolerable

burning in urethra, with chordee (painful erection of penis).
4. Erythema from exposure to sun-rays.
5. Vesicular erysipelas; vesicles all over the body are sore and suppurating (pus-forming).
6. Inflammations rapidly developing into gangrene (dead tissue).
7. *Hydrophobia* : Renewal of convulsions at the sight of dazzling objects or water.
8. Stoppage of urine in cholera.
9. Retention of placenta.
10. Puerperal (after-delivery) mania—sexual type.
11. Sudden loss of consciousness with red face.
12. Promotes fecundity and expulsions of moles, placenta, dead foetus and foreign bodies from uterus.

Note :- If skin is broken, alcoholic preparations should not be used; dilutions in warm water promptly relieves the burning and the pain.

## 14. CARBO VEGETABILIS
### (Carb-v.)

1. Collapsing condition with coldness, sweating, pale face, feeble pulse, cold tongue, cold breath, cyanosis (skin blue from deoxygenated blood) needing oxygen, wants to be fanned.
2. Shock after surgical operation, trauma, electric shock, allergic or due to acute and serious diseases, cold body, pale face, cold breath; perspires profusely and wants to be fanned.
3. Passive haemorrhages in delicate and feeble persons.
4. Fainting in anaemic and debilitated persons.
5. Bad effects from fatty, rich food, alcohol, wine, debauchery, putrid fish or meat.
6. Acute diseases, e.g., pneumonia, bronchitis, dyspnoea (difficult breathing) in old persons.

7. Metastasis (transfer) of mumps to mammae or testicles.
8. Bad effects of some exhausting illness.
9. Asthma from measles or pertussis (whooping cough) of childhood.
10. Remote effects of injuries received long ago.
11. Ulcers or other diseases taking a chronic course, after bad effects of typhoid, or typhus.
12. Bad effects of mercury or quinine, suppressed malaria.
13. **Most suitable for:**
    (a) premature persons enfeebled by acute diseases;
    (b) old persons with feeble circulation;
    (c) women at the turn of life, i.e., menopause;
    (d) who are susceptible to warm and wet weather;
    (e) who are sensitive to any irregularity in their diet;
    (f) who are of scorbutic (affected with scurvy), flatulent (gas-forming) and allergic disposition;
    (g) chronic diseases in persons of low vitality due to lack of reaction;
    (h) weak persons with low vitality due to loss of blood.

## 15. CHAMOMILLA
### (Cham.)

1. Diarrhoea of nursing children; stools green, watery, corroding and offensive.
2. Diarrhoea of children during dentition.
3. Toothache worse from warm applications.
4. Convulsions during dentition.
5. Violent rheumatic pains drive him out of bed at night, compel him to walk about.
6. Patient cannot endure anyone near him, is cross, cannot bear to be spoken to, averse to talking; answers peevishly, is oversensitive to pain; pain drives him to despair, aggravated by heat; great aversion to wind and open air;

sleepy but cannot sleep; burning soles at night, puts feet out of bed.
7. Convulsions of children from nursing after a fit of anger in mother.
8. Infantile earache.
9. **Most suitable for :**
    (a) children who are exceedingly irritable, peevish, fretful, snappish; cannot return a civil answer; are quiet only when carried; want this or that and become angry when refused, or when offered, petulently reject it; too ugly to live, are cross and spiteful;
    (b) in cases spoiled by the use of opium or morphine; in complaints of children.

**Note:** Mental calmness contra-indicates *Chamomilla*.

## 16. COCCULUS INDICUS
### (Cocc.)

1. Motion sickness, as from travelling in a motor car, boat or rail-road transport, etc.; acts as a prophylactic, if taken for two days before the trip in 30th potency.
2. Bad effects of loss of sleep.
3. Bad effects of continued worry and anxiety, anger, grief.
4. Vomiting of pregnancy with vertigo.
5. Diphtheritic paralysis; paralysis of throat, lower extremities. Paralysis after septic conditions.
6. Ailments of drunkards.
7. Hernia with incarcerated flatulence (confined gas), especially umbilical, when *Nux-v.* fails.
8. The thought and smell of food will nauseate the patient (*Ars.*).
9. Mental derangements with vertigo.
10. Exhausting menses, scarcely able to speak.

## 17. COLOCYNTHIS
### (Colo.)

1. Neuralgic (nerve) pains better from pressure and heat.
2. Pains of iris and glaucoma (hardness of eyeball leading to blindness), when they extend to the head and are better by pressure.
3. *Sciatica :* Shooting pain, lightning-like shocks, down the whole left lower extremity, left hip, left thigh, left knee into popliteal fossa (depression on thigh bone near knee); crampy pain in hip, as though screwed in a vice; lies upon the affected side; better from heat and pressure.
4. *Colic :* Better from bending double or pressing something hard against the abdomen; from anger; from eating cheese; from gastric disorders; griping pains; spasmodic pain; alternates with vertigo; with cramps in calves; with diarrhoea; worse at night and after eating.
5. Diarrhoea from grief, indignation or anger.
6. Diabetes with milky, gelatinous or colloid (glutinous) urine.
7. *Ailments from anger*: Colic, diarrhoea, suppressed lochia, vomiting, suppressed menses.
8. Ailments in extremely irritable and impatient persons, who become angry or are offended on being questioned; irritable; throw things away out of the hand.

## 18. CUPRUM METALLICUM
### (Cupr.)

1. Cholera, with cramps in abdomen and calves.
2. *Whooping cough :* long-lasting, suffocating, spasmodic cough, causing breathlessness, blue face and rigid, stiff body.
3. *Convulsions,* with blue face and clenched thumbs.
4. *Cramps* in extremities, with great weariness of limbs.

5. Cough has a gurgling sound, as if water was being poured from a bottle; cough better by drinking cold water.
6. *Epilepsy*: Aura begins in knees and ascends.
7. While drinking, the fluid descends with a gurgling sound.
8. A strong, sweetish, metallic, coppery taste in the mouth with flow of saliva.
9. Paralysis of tongue; imperfect, stammering speech.
10. *Spasms* : Beginning in fingers and toes, and spreading over the whole body.
11. Bad effects of fright, over-exertion and loss of sleep.
12. Suppressed foot sweats, discharges.

## 19. EUPHRASIA
### (Euphr.)

1. Ailments with acrid (biting) lachrymation and bland coryza, influenza, measles, headache, blepharitis (inflamed eyelids), acute conjunctivitis; prostatic troubles, Third nerve paralysis; amenorrhoea; whooping cough.
2. *Eye affections* : Staphyloma (protrusion of cornea or sclera of eye), pannus, granular lids, catarrhal conjunctivitis, corneal ulcers, iritis, ptosis (drooping eyelids).
3. Measles with acrid lachrymation and bland coryza.
4. Cancer of the nose.
5. Falls, injuries.
6. Nasal catarrh, with lachrymation.

## 20. FERRUM PHOSPHORICUM
### (Ferr-p.)

1. First stage of all inflammatory affections.
2. Bright red haemorrhages from any orifice.

3. Congestive headache, vertigo, sore throat, relief from cold applications.
4. Fever due to congestion, heat of sun or mechanical injuries.
5. Acute otitis media (ear inflammation).
6. *Cerebral Haemorrhage*: Face pale and flushed alternately; mucous membranes pale; pulse rapid and thready; in anaemic persons.

## 21. GELSEMIUM
### (Gels.)

It is a **polycrest remedy** (having many uses) frequently used in acute diseases. It is not a deep acting remedy and, therefore, it is followed by deep acting remedies in chronic diseases.

**It is a constitutional remedy** for children, young boys and girls, nervous men and women, highly emotional, hysterical, fearful, timid, apprehensive people and those who lack vital force due to self-abuse or alcohol.

**It is a specific remedy** for mental disorders, brain diseases, nervous diseases, paralysis, eye diseases, deafness, fevers, neuralgias, hay fever, jaundice, rheumatism, vertigo, headache, angina pectoris and heart disorders, drooping of eyelids, menstrual disorders and male sex disorders; when the guiding characteristic symptoms general characteristic symptoms are present or when the history of causation is present.

Following are the **leading symptoms** for the use of *Gelsemium*.

1. Complete relaxation and prostration of whole muscular system, with entire motor (movement) paralysis.
2. The anticipation of any unusual ordeal, preparing for church, theatre or to meet an engagement brings on diarrhoea.
3. Stage fright; nervous dread of appearing in public.
4. General depression from heat of sun or summer.

5. Weakness and trembling; lack of muscular coordination; the muscles do not obey the will.
6. Vertigo, spreading from the occiput, with dim vision and feeling as if intoxicated.
7. Headache beginning in the nape of neck (occiput) and extending over the head; worse by mental exertion, smoking, heat of sun and lying with head low, and better by profuse urination.
8. Chill without thirst, especially along the spine, running up and down the back.
9. The patient is dull, drowsy and dizzy.

## 22. GLONOINE
### (Glon.)

1. *Cerebral Haemorrhage:* Violent palpitation of heart which is visible as shaking the chest; restlessness and twitching of muscles.
2. *Epilepsy:* Aura, violent, pulsating headache, worse in warm room, before the fit, followed by unconsciousness. Face is pale and bright red by turns. Throbbing of heart-beat felt all over the body, especially the head.
3. *Sunstroke:* with violent headache; pounding sensation with every heart-beat; grasps the head with his hands to stop pounding; worse by shaking the head and by stooping.
4. *Vertigo:* With pulsating pain in head; with flushing of face; intoxicated feeling and fainting; vertigo caused by shaking the head; worse from stooping.
5. *Headache:* From heat of the sun or working under gaslight; menstrual; climacteric (menopausal); from acute congestion of head, bursting; throbbing; pulsating; holds head with both hands; worse from lying down; after profuse uterine haemorrhage; in place of menses; worse from jar and stooping.

6. *Thermic Fever:* From excessive heat of the sun; face pale with high fever; head hot and extremities cold; with beating of carotid and templar (neck and head) arteries; with cerebral congestion. Cerebro-spinal fever.
7. *Convulsions:* During dentition (*Bell., Cham.*), from cerebral congestion.
8. *Exophthalmic Goitre:* With carotid pulsation or violent palpitation; with bursting headache; with rush of blood to the face.
9. *Angina Pectoris*: Sharp pains in heart with laboured action; throbbing in carotids; blood seems to rush to heart and rapidly to head.
10. Bad effects of mental excitement, fright, fear, causing palpitation; headache, sleeplessness.

## 23. HEPAR SULPHURIS
### (Hep. Sulph.)

1. *Syphilitic Affections*: When mercury has been abused; when there is offensive odour from the mouth of the patient suffering from syphilitic affections of mouth, nose and throat; primary chancre (hard swelling), suppuration of buboes and gummas (hard and soft swellings), with foetid and purulent discharge.
2. *Croup*: From exposure to dry cold wind; worse in morning and evening, until midnight; barking cough with hoarseness and rattling of mucus; worse from cold air, cold drinks; better from warmth.
3. *Asthma*: After suppressed eruption; wheezing, rattling and threatened suffocation.
4. *Ailments*: With profuse, sour, offensive perspiration; worse from lying on painful side; cold air; uncovering; eating and drinking cold things; better from warmth, wrapping the head and in damp wet weather.

5. **Especially adapted to the following types of patients:**
   (a) who are extremely susceptible and sensitive to cold; chilly; who cannot tolerate the air if the door is opened; cannot bear to be uncovered; take cold from slightest exposure to fresh air;
   (b) who are over-sensitive; the slightest cause irritates; cannot tolerate pain, which causes fainting; the skin is very sensitive to touch, cannot bear even clothes touching the affected parts;
   (c) patients who are peevish, angry at the least trifle; hypochondriacal (morbid anxiety about health); unreasonably anxious; oversensitive to persons and to places;
   (d) patients, who are highly impulsive; sudden impulses crop up; it becomes a mania to set fire to things;
   (e) persons with tendency to suppuration (pus formation) in parts of the body; with irritability of temper; suppurative tonsillitis, otitis medial, corneal ulcers, leucorrhoea, whitlow, suppuration in the bones, necrosis and caries (tissue or bone degeneration).

## 24. HYPERICUM PERFORATUM
### (Hyper.)

1. *Excessive painfulness:* In crushed fingers; punctured, gunshot, lacerated, incised wounds; after operations or amputations.
2. Preserves integrity of torn and lacerated tissues when almost entirely separated from the body.
3. Injuries to spinal cord; concussions; pain after a fall on coccyx; lumbar puncture; convulsions after injury to head. *Hypericum* removes pain and their bad effects.
4. Removes nervous depression following wounds or surgical operations.
5. Removes pain and bad effects of rat bite; nerve injuries.

7. Prevents tetanus after traumatic injuries.
8. Arrests ulceration and sloughing of wounds.
9. Removes headache after a fall on occiput, especially when the patient feels as if being lifted up high into the air.
10. *Asthma* from foggy weather.
11. Piles bleeding and excessively painful.
12. Toothache; bunions and corns when pain is excruciating due to involvement of nerves.

## 25. IPECACUANHA
### (Ipecac.)

1. *Asthma :* Violent attacks; with constriction in chest, wheezing cough, suffocation, dyspnoea (breathlessness). One of the first remedies in an acute attack.
2. *Malarial fever*: With persistent nausea and vomiting, periodical attacks; suppressed by quinine. Dumb ague.
3. *Haemorrhages*: Epistaxis, haematemesis (blood vomiting), haemorrhoidal, menstrual; profuse; of bright red colour; sudden, violent.
4. Dysentery with nausea and vomiting; with green mucus and blood; in autumn; when the nights are cold and days hot.
5. Cholera; when the prominent symptoms are nausea and vomiting.
6. *Whooping cough*: convulsive or spasmodic, with rigidity; with nausea and vomiting; bleeding from nose or mouth.
7. Gallstone colic with nausea, retching and vomiting, cutting, flatulent colic about umbilicus (navel). Colic from cold drinks or ice cream.
8. Hoarseness and Aphonia (voice lost) after an attack of cold.
9. Granulations (growths) of the lids have been cured by the instillation of the dilutions.
10. It is an **antidote** to **Morphia habit,** when given in drop doses.

## 26. LACHESIS
### (Lach.)

1. *Diphtheria*: Left-sided, goes from left to right side; in warm-blooded persons, worse in warm room and by hot drinks; with dark purple appearance of the throat; worse after sleep; intolerance of any tight clothing around the neck.
2. *Fevers*: Typhoid, typhus, malaria, septic; returning annually or in spring or summer; with stupor or muttering delirium; tongue trembles when protruded; conjuctiva (membrane covering eyeball) yellow or orange colour; perspiration cold, yellow staining.
3. Bad effects of poisonous wounds, post-mortem room wounds; suppressed discharges, coryza, menses; alcohol, mercury, cinchona, acids.
4. Ailments from sun's rays, spring, summer, onanism (interrupted coition), jealousy, emotions.
5. Diseases begin on left side and go to the right side; left ovary, left testicle, left throat, left chest, left eye, etc.
6. Ailments with dark, bluish, purple appearance, tend to malignancy; boils, carbuncles, ulcers with much pain, bed-sores, malignant pustules.
7. *Epilepsy*: Comes on during sleep; from loss of vital fluids, onanism, jealousy.
8. Climacteric (menopausal) ailments with rush of blood to head; intolerance of tight clothes about neck or waist; great sensitiveness to touch.
9. Ailments, worse after sleep, or aggravation wakes him from sleep, with great loquacity; constipation without urging; pains relieved by flow of menses; great mental and physical exhaustion; rush of blood to head; weight and pressure on vertex, like lead in occiput.
10. *Piles*: Strangulated; with stitches shooting upward; with scanty menses.
11. **Especially adapted to patients who are :**
    (a) warm-blooded who are worse in summer, from sun's rays, hot drinks and in a warm room;

(b) susceptible to emotions — grief, sorrow, fright, vexation, jealousy, disappointed love;
(c) disposed to haemorrhagic diathesis (predisposition), apoplexy, erysipelas, climacteric disturbances;
(d) having a broken-down constitution.

## 27. LEDUM PALUSTRE
(Led.)

1. *Black Eye*: Ecchymosis (discolouration) of lids and conjunctiva, injury to eye with a blunt weapon; boxing or blow on the eye.
2. Haemorrhage into anterior chamber of eye after iridotomy (incision in iris).
3. Punctured wounds by a needle, nail, awl or any sharp instrument.
4. Insect-bite from bees, wasps, mosquitoes, scorpions; rat or cat-bite.
5. Long remaining discolouration after injuries; black or blue.
6. Easy spraining of ankles and feet.
7. *Gout*: Begins in lower limbs and ascends; joints become seat of nodosities (swellings) and "gout stone", which are painful.
8. *Rheumatism*: pains are sticking, tearing, throbbing; worse by motion; at night; by warmth of bed and covering (*Merc. Puls.*); better or relieved by holding feet in ice water (*Puls.*). Affects left shoulder and right hip-joint.
9. Ball of toes painful, swollen; tendon stiff, worse on stepping and walking. Pain in heels as if bruised.
10. *Swelling*: of feet upto knees; of ankle, as from a sprain or false step.
11. **Especially suited to the following types of patients:**
    (a) who are full-blooded and Plethoric, of a robust character, with red face, and are fleshy and strongly built; predisposed to haemorrhages;

- (b) who are chilly during acute diseases; lack of animal or vital heat; feel cold all the time;
- (c) though parts are cold to touch but not cold subjectively to the patient;
- (d) broken-down constitutions by alcohol; with craving for whisky.

## 28. LYCOPODIUM CLAVATUM
### (Lyco.)

1. Ailments: affecting right side or extending from right to left side; worse from 4 to 8 p.m.; better from warm food and drinks; from uncovering the head; must loosen the garments; deep-seated, progressive, chronic diseases; with canine hunger; headache, if he does not eat.
2. Ailments from fright, anger, mortification, vexation, with reserved displeasure.
3. Impotency in young men from onanism (unnatural sex) or sexual excesses.
4. Bad effects of onions, bread, wine, spirituous liquors, tobacco smoking and chewing.
5. *Diphtheria*: Right-sided; goes from right to left; descends from nose to right tonsil; worse after sleep and from cold drinks.
6. *Catarrh*: Dry nasal; nose stopped at night, must breathe through the mouth; snuffles (nasal discharge); child starts from sleep rubbing his nose; catarrh of root of nose and frontal sinuses; with formation of crusts and elastic plugs.
7. *Malarial fever* : With sour vomiting between chill and heat.
8. *Acid Dyspepsia* with sour eructations, heartburn, waterbrash and sour vomiting.
9. *Flatulence*: Excessive; fullness not relieved by belching; a few mouthfuls fill up to the throat, and he feels bloated; distension, especially in lower abdomen.

10. *Renal colic* right-sided, with flatulence and constipation; pain in back relieved by urination; red sand in urine; in irritable, fearful people who desire company.

11. Pneumonia with fan-like motion of *alae nasi* (flaps of the nose); twitching of forehead, affecting base of right lung and difficult expectoration; neglected or maltreated.

12. Hernia right-sided, especially in children.

13. **Especially suitable for:**

    (a) infants — baby cries all the day, sleeps all night; constipated; red sand on child's diaper; child cries before urinating;

    (b) children — weak, emaciated; with well-developed head but puny sickly bodies; waking at night feeling hungry; irritable; peevish and cross on waking; ugly, kicking and screaming; easily angered; cannot endure opposition or contradiction; seek disputes; are beside themselves;

    (c) women — weep all the day, cannot calm themselves; very sensitive; even cry when thanked; constipation since puberty; since last confinement; dryness of vagina; burning during and after coition; physometra (air in uterine cavity); foetus appears to be turning somersaults;

    (d) men — dread of other men, of solitude; fear of being alone; irritable and melancholic; avaricious, greedy, miserly, malicious, pusillanimous (easily fightened) Complexion pale, dirty, unhealthy, sallow, with deep furrows, looks older than he is; impotency of young men, from sexual excess; penis small, cold, relaxed; old men with strong desire but imperfect erections; falls asleep during an embrace; premature emissions;

    (e) extremes of life, children and old people; predisposed to lung and liver affections.

## 29. MAGNESIA PHOSPHORICA
### (Mag-p.)

1. Affections of right side of the body — head, ear, face, chest, ovary, sciatic nerve.
2. Ailments of teething children; spasms or convulsions without fever.
3. Headache begins in occiput and extends over to head; of schoolgirls; face red, flushed; from mental, emotional exertion or hard study; worse 10 to 11 a.m. or 4 to 5 p.m.; better from warmth and pressure.
4. Neuralgia of face, supra- or infra-orbital (above and below eye socket); right-sided; intermittent, darting, cutting; worse from cold air; better from warmth and pressure.
5. Toothache during night; rapidly shifting; worse from eating, drinking, especially cold things; better from warmth and pressure.
6. Pains sharp, cutting, stabbing; shooting, stitching, lightning-like in coming and going; intermittent, paroxysms becoming almost unbearable, driving patient to frenzy; rapidly changing place; with constricting sensation; cramping; in neuralgic affections of stomach, abdomen and pelvis.
7. Spasms or cramps of stomach, with clean tongue; as if a band was drawn tightly around the body.
8. Colic flatulent, forcing patient to bend double; better from warmth, pressure and rubbing; of cows and horses, when *Colo.* fails.
9. Dysmenorrhoea (menstrual pain) worse before menses; better after flow; pains darting like lightning, shooting; right-sided; better from warmth and pressure.
10. Cramps of extremities; during pregnancy; of writers, piano or violin players.
11. **Especially adapted to those:**
    (a) who are thin, emaciated and highly nervous;
    (b) who are chilly; are afraid of cold air, cold bathing and uncovering; are worse from cold air, cold draught, cold bathing and washing; better from warmth and pressure;
    (c) who are languid, tired, exhausted; unable to sit.

## 30. MERCURIUS SOLUBILIS
### (Merc.)

1. Abscess, aphthous stomatitis (sore mouth), balanitis (inflammation of glans penis), bone diseases, bubo, chicken-pox, chancre, colds, condylomata (wart-like growths near ankles or vulva)—syphilitic or gonorrhoeal, catarrh, dentitional troubles, diarrhoea, dysentery, dyspepsia, glandular swellings, gout, gum-boil, heat affections, herpes, jaundice, lumbago, measles, phimosis (tightness of foreskin of penis), pregnancy disorders, scurvy, small-pox, throat troubles, toothache, tremors, ulcers.

2. *Toothache*: Pulsating; shooting into face or ear; worse from cold water; worse at night with profuse salivation and spongy gums.

3. Cough dry and fatiguing, racking; in two paroxysms, worse at night; in the warmth of bed and lying on right side.

4. Diarrhoea of infants, green stools; slimy and offensive; excoriating the anus.

5. Dysentery acute; stools bloody, slimy, greenish; with pain and tenesmus; never get done feeling; with cutting colic; worse at night.

6. Coryza with sneezing; raw, smarting sensation, profuse, fluent; worse damp weather.

7. *Fever:* Great thirst with moist mouth; profuse perspiration without relief; worse at night; in warm room and warm bed.

8. Whooping cough with nose-bleed.

9. *Syphilis*: Iritis; ulcers; primary and secondary syphilis with glandular enlargements; bone-pains; worse at night and damp weather.

10. Infective Hepatitis : Fever with profuse perspiration which does not relieve but aggravates; with jaundice; excessive salivation with thirst; worse lying on right side;

sensitive to both heat and cold. Icterus neonatorum (jaundice in the new-born).

11. Paralysis agitans (shaking paralysis), chorea, Parkinsonian disease, tremors and nervous debility.

12. Otitis (ear inflammation) with thick yellow, foetid discharge; ruptured drum; worse at night and warmth of bed.

13. Leucorrhoea acrid, burning, itching; with rawness; pruritus (itching) worse from contact of urine, which must be washed off. Specific or non-specific vaginitis (inflammation of vagina) with greenish excoriating discharge.

14. *Urinary troubles*: Constant desire, but little urine passed; must urinate at least every hour, day and night, with burning in urethra on beginning to urinate; urine passes involuntarily if he does not hurry.

15. It has affinity for diseases of glandular organs; parotids, tonsils, liver, spleen and kidneys; worse at night and warmth of bed; with excessive salivation; tongue having imprints of teeth.

16. **Especially adapted to the following types of patients:**

    (a) who are susceptible to cold damp weather;

    (b) who are sensitive to both cold and heat;

    (c) who are aggravated from lying on right side;

    (d) who have profuse salivation, wet the pillow in sleep; show imprints of teeth on the tongue; tongue is large and flabby;

    (e) who have odour from mouth and body;

    (f) who perspire easily and perspiration aggravates their symptoms;

    (g) who suffer from great weakness and trembling from least exertion;

    (h) who have a combination of the above symptoms.

## 31. NUX VOMICA
### (Nux-v.)

1. Ailments from bad effects of coffee, alcohol, tobacco, spicy food, over-eating, loss of sleep.
2. Convulsions with consciousness; worse from anger, emotions, touch and moving.
3. Pains are tingling, sticking, aching, worse from motion and contact.
4. Fever with severe chill, must be covered in every stage of fever; chill is worse from motion.
5. Strangulated umbilical hernia of infants and children.
6. Snuffles of infants; stoppage of nose.
7. Constipation; with frequent unsuccessful desire; sensation as if not finished.
8. Menses irregular, never at right time; every two weeks; stopping and starting again.
9. Labour pains violent, spasmodic; cause fainting, urging to defecate or urinate.
10. **One of the best remedies with which to commence treatment in those who are drugged by hot and strong medicines.**
11. It is a remedy *par excellence* for the following types of patients:
    (a) **who are OVERSENSITIVE** : Oversensitive to noise, light, touch, cold air, surroundings, food, spices, rich food, hot food, over-eating, tea, coffee, narcotics, allopathic medicines, wine, alcoholic preparations;
    (b) who are **IRRITABLE**, touchy, offended even by harmless words; inclination to commit suicide, but are afraid to die; easily excited or angered; cannot bear contradiction; trifling ailments and pains are unbearable;
    (c) who are sedentary in habits (physical idleness), undergo mental exertion; loss of sleep; anxious, full of worries;
    (d) who are chilly, always taking cold which extends from nose to chest, worse from draught of cold air; worse

from uncovering; must be covered in every stage of fever;

(e) who have a tendency to faint: from odours; after eating; after every labour pain; in the morning.

## 32. PHOSPHORUS
### (Phos.)

1. *Constipation*: Faeces slender, long, dry, tough and hard; voided with great straining and difficulty.
2. *Diarrhoea* watery with sago-like particles; anus remains open; involuntary; during cholera time; morning; old man's diarrhoea; during menses.
3. *Cough* on going from warm to cold air; worse from laughing, talking, reading, drinking, eating, lying on left side.
4. *Haemorrhage*: Metrorrhagia (abnormal uterine bleeding), haemoptysis (blood spitting), epistaxis, haematemesis, vicarious menses; from urethra and anus; metrorrhagia with cancer of uterus, frequent and profuse with ringing in ears, fainting, loss of sight, general coldness, sometimes with convulsions. Haemorrhagic diathesis; small wounds bleed much. After tooth-extraction. Epistaxis in children who grow up too rapidly.
5. Tubercular deposits begin in apex of lung, usually on the left side.
6. *Ailments* after loss of vital fluids; which are worse lying on left side, and before and during thunderstorm; with all gone sensation in abdomen, relieved by eating; with burning pains in small spots; with complaints that appear diagonally, upper right, lower left; with vomiting of water as soon as it reaches the stomach, desire for cold water.
7. Aphonia from singing; hoarseness, worse in the evening.
8. Pain in the chest, intercostal spaces (between ribs), worse from slightest pressure and lying on left side; excited by cold air.

9. Necrosis (tissue death) of the left lower jaw.
10. Fevers with great desire for cold drinks, juicy, refreshing things; ice-cream which relieves gastric pains.
11. *Nasal polypus*: Bleeding profusely.
12. *Eye diseases*: Blindness due to sexual excesses; retinitis, simple or albuminurous; detachment of retina; retinal apoplexy and muscular asthenopia (tiring with pain, etc.).
13. **Especially suited to the following types of patients:**
    (a) who are born sick, feeble, anaemic, nervous, want to be magnetised;
    (b) who grow up too rapidly, slender, fair skin, delicate, fine blonde or red hair;
    (c) who have quick perception, very sensitive to external impressions, light, noise, odours, touch;
    (d) who are restless, fidgety, move continually, cannot stand or sit still for a moment, are inclined to stoop, and suffer from nervous tremblings;
    (e) who are weak and easily exhausted, weary of life, full of gloomy forebodings;
    (f) who have a weak, empty, all-gone sensation in head, chest, stomach and entire abdomen; who have longing for acids, spicy things, ice-creams and very cold water;
    (g) who have haemorrhagic diathesis (predisposition); small wounds bleed profusely from every mucous outlet;
    (h) who are disposed to phthisis;
    (i) old people with morning diarrhoea.

## 33. PLANTAGO MAJOR
(Plant.)

1. Periodical prosopalgia (facial pain), worse from 7 a.m. to 2 p.m., with flow of tears, photophobia; pains radiate to temples and lower face.

2. Sharp pain in the eyes, reflex from decayed teeth or inflammation of middle ear; pain plays between teeth and ears.
3. *Earache*: Pain goes from one ear to the other through the head; saliva flows with the pains.
4. *Otalgia* (earache), with toothache; loud noises go through one.
5. Toothache which is sensitive and sore to least touch; feels too prolonged; worse night, cold air and contact, better for sleep and while eating; pyorrhoea; profuse flow of saliva.
6. Nocturnal enuresis (bed-wetting), polyuria (excessive urine).

## 34. PULSATILLA
### (Puls.)

1. *Diarrhoea*: Only or usually at night; as soon as they eat; from fruits, impure water, cold food or drinks; no two stools alike; changeable.
2. *Styes*: Especially on upper lid; from eating fat, rich food or pork.
3. *Toothache:* Worse from warm things and heat of the room; relieved by holding cold water in the mouth (*Bry.*); during pregnancy.
4. *Metastasis* (transfer) of mumps to testicles or mammary glands.
5. Gonorrhoeal orchitis (inflammation of testicles); rheumatism; stricture of urethra, urine passes only in drops.
6. Ailments from fats, rich food, fruits, getting feet wet, suppressed menses, exposure to cold, pregnancy.
7. **Otalgia** (earache) worse at night; better from cold applications.
8. Sub-acute conjunctivitis with dyspepsia; worse in warm room.

9. *Dysentery* with mucus and blood, with chilliness; no two stools alike.
10. *Cough* from fatty food; urine emitted with cough; after measles.
11. *Urticaria* after rich food; from delayed menses; worse undressing; with diarrhoea.
12. Malarial fever with absence of thirst in all stages; one-sided sweats.
13. Catarrhal conjunctivitis, worse from warm applications and better from cold applications.
14. Incontinence of urine in young girls who have leucorrhoea; the desire comes on suddenly and they wet their clothes or bed; urine is turbid.
15. Hydrocele with *Pulsatilla* temperament and characteristic symptoms.
16. Incipient tuberculosis with delayed menses; with cough and loss of weight.
17. Sterility due to profuse chronic leucorrhoea.
18. Phantom pregnancy; woman imagines that she is pregnant, with other symptoms of *Puls*.
19. **One of the best remedies to begin with in the treatment of a chronic case.**
20. Asthma of children who are allergic to fats, rich food, fruits.
21. Asthma of women with irregular menses.
22. Ailments with chill, weeping easily, thick and bland discharges, changing or contradictory symptoms; worse in evening, and lying on left side; thirstlessness; desires cool open air.
23. **Chronic nasal catarrh**: Discharge thick yellow, greenish, offensive.
24. It is especially suited to the following **types of patients**:
    (a) children: with pale face, blue eyes, liking fun and

caresses; weepy; want company; averse to warmth; no two stools alike;

(b) girls: fleshy, affectionate, mild, gentle, timid; weep easily; with scanty, delayed menses; derangements at puberty; feel uncomfortable in warm and closed room, better in open air. Epilepsy with absence or irregularity of menses; milk in breasts from tight clothings;

(c) women: weep while giving out symptoms to the doctor; like company and consolation; symptoms ever changing, must have fresh air; threatened abortion, flow ceases and then returns with increased force; pains spasmodic, excite suffocation and fainting; suppressed menses from wet feet; intermittent, changeable and clotted; chilliness attended with menses; leucorrhoea acrid, excoriating, and burning; diarrhoea during or after menses. Helps in normalising the malposition of foetus and spurious labour pains; useful in complaints of pregnancy, like vomiting, diarrhoea, heartburn and bladder troubles; retained placenta;

(d) patients: anaemic, chlorotic (with greenish pallor of skin), who have taken much iron, quinine and tonics, even years before; who are badly affected by taking rich, fatty, indigestible food; worse in the evening at twilight; who feel chilly in warm room, awake unrefreshed after sleep; the first serious impairment of health is referred to puberty, "never been well since" — anaemia, chlorosis, bronchitis; phthisis; symptoms ever changing; pains rapidly shifting from one part to another; pains attended with chilliness; the more severe the pain, the more severe the chill; pains appear suddenly and leave gradually; thirstlessness with nearly all complaints; great dryness of mouth in the morning without thirst; all gone sensation in stomach in tea drinkers; discharges thick, bland and yellowish green; want head high on two pillows; lie with hands above head; worse from letting the affected limb hang down.

## 35. RHUS TOXICODENDRON
### (Rhus-t.)

1. *Fever*: Typhoid, Dengue fever, Erysipelas, Influenza, Pleurisy, Measles, Pneumonia, Septicaemia, Scarlet fever, rheumatic fever, Typhus fever with restlessness, soreness, stiffness, lameness; must change position to obtain relief from soreness or pain; fever blisters around mouth; tongue dry, sore, red at the tip, takes imprint of teeth; low muttering delirium, great apprehension at night; fears he will die of being poisoned; thirst for water; dry teasing cough, worse from exposure to cold and wet weather; lying quietly; better from warmth, wrapping up warmly; cough during chill.

2. *Ailments* from spraining, straining, over-stretching, over-lifting; lying on damp ground; too much summer bathing in lake or river.

3. *Paralysis* with numbness of the affected parts; from damp and cold; after exertion; after delivery; sexual excesses; typhoid; paresis (paralysis) of limbs; ptosis (drooping, particularly of eyelids) with loss of sensation; right-sided hemiplegia (paralysis); infantile paralysis.

4. Prolapse of uterus from over-reaching or straining.

5. Tonsillitis after riding in cold wind (*Acon., Hep.*).

6. *Urticaria* after bathing; with fever; with intolerable itching, worse from cold air; with rheumatic complaints.

7. Cerebro-spinal meningitis with anxiety and restlessness.

8. Diarrhoea in typhoid fever; worse during night; better during day.

9. Hoarseness on first beginning to sing, which wears off after singing for a while.

10. Hypertrophy of heart from violent exercise; gets out of breath on exertion.

11. Eczema capitis (on scalp) of infants; dry, itchy eruptions; worse in winter, cold wet weather, with intolerable itching in bed during night.

12. Herpes zoster with *Rhus-tox.* characteristic symptoms.
13. Sprains of ankle with oedema.
14. Diphtheria with *Rhus-tox.* symptoms.
15. **It is an excellent remedy for the following types of patients:**
    (a) who are susceptible to cold, wet environments, wearing wet shirts, socks, lying on damp ground or wet sheets; suffer from stiffness, pains or paralytic symptoms;
    (b) persons of rheumatic diathesis; muscular rheumatism, fibrositis (inflammatory increase of white tissue fibres), iritis, stiffness of jaws, crackling in the articulation of jaw when moving it; rheumatic heart with sticking pains with lameness and numbness of left arm; stiffness of neck with painful tension; aching in small of back while sitting, relieved by continuous motion; dull aching pain in right sciatic nerve; stiffness of knees; rheumatic inflammation of joints from exposure to cold and damp weather, amelioration from heat, rubbing, continuous motion; with great restlessness, soreness and stiffness.

## 36. RUTA GRAVEOLENS
### (Ruta)

1. Lameness after sprains, especially of wrists and ankles.
2. Eye troubles; from over-exertion of eyes; over-use in bad light, over-reading at night; fine sewing, watch-repairing; anomalies of refraction; asthenopia (weakness of eyes with pain, etc.); burning in eyes like balls of fire; congestion of eyes, spasms of lower lids; paralytic weakness; strabismus (squint); amblyopia (dimness of vision); blurred vision, aching in and over eyes
3. Phthisis after mechanical injuries to chest; haemoptysis (blood spitting), with hacking cough.

4. After a fall bruised sensation all over the body, especially limbs and joints; the parts laid upon are painful; must change the position.
5. Constipation from inactivity, or impaction (firmly lodged stools) following mechanical injuries.
6. Prolapse of rectum on passing stools; after confinement; aggravated by stooping; preceding a very difficult stool.
7. Injured and bruised bones.
8. Cancer of rectum.
9. Backache, ameliorated by lying on back; pressure; sitting after a long walk; rest and continued motion (*Rhus-t.*).
10. Sore and sensitive nodes in bones and tendons of muscles after injury.
11. Knees give way going up or down stairs.
12. *Warts*: Flat smooth on palms with sore pains.
13. *Sciatica*: Aggravated on lying at night; better in the day on moving.
14. Urticaria from eating meat.
15. Ganglion (cystic tumour) on wrist.

## 37. SPIGELIA
### (Spig.)

1. *Worm affections* of scrofulous children, who refer to the navel as the most painful part; eye complaints with worm troubles; headache, neuralgias, itching at anus, foetid breath, cardiac symptoms or stammering with worm troubles.
2. *Neuralgia*: Left-sided; from cold damp weather; prosopalgia (faceache), periodical, in orbit, eye, malar bone, teeth; from morning until sunset; pains tearing, burning; cheek dark red.
3. *Rheumatism*: Pain in knees with heart symptoms.
4. Glaucoma of left eye.

5. Exophthalmic goitre with palpitation.
6. Stammering, repeats first syllable three or four times, with worm or abdominal troubles; makes great efforts to speak; distorts the face.
7. *Dyspnoea* (difficult breathing): Must lie on right side with head high.
8. Toothache from tobacco-smoking, better while eating, lying down; worse from cold air or water.
9. *Palpitation*: Violent, visible, audible; from least motion; when bending forward; systolic blowing at apex.
10. Cancerous rectum or sigmoid colon with atrocious unbearable pains.
11. *Angina Pectoris*: Worse from motion; chest pains are stitching, worse from cold air or cold wet weather.
12. Contraction of fingers (*Gels.*).
13. Neuralgia before eruptions of Herpes zoster.
14. Occipital (back portion) headache, spreads over the head and settles over left eye.

## 38. SPONGIA TOSTA
### (Spong.)

1. *Heart troubles* : Associated with palpitation, dyspnoea, marked anxiety, fear of death; waking up suddenly at night in fright with suffocation and being unable to lie down on bed; cardiac dyspnoea, worse lying down, warm room, better from warm drinks; rheumatic endocarditis (inflammation of heart covering) with hypertrophy (enlargement) of heart; angina pectoris worse from ascending, motion, at night.
2. *Severe forms of Asthma*: With dryness of respiratory passages; dry throat, dry larynx, dry trachea and dry bronchi; seldom rattling; whistling and wheezing; at times great dyspnoea, difficult expectoration, which has to be swallowed; with headache; bending forward ameliorates.

3. *Goitre, Hyperthyroidism* (excess functioning of thyroid gland): Eyes protruding with heart symptoms; with palpitation, dyspnoea on exertion, with contracting pains, faintness, anxiety, worse in warm room; suffocative paroxysms at night.
4. Sore throat after eating sweet things.
5. *Croup*: With anxiety, wheezing, worse during inspiration; worse at midnight, no exudation, but infiltration.
6. *Cough*: Dry, barking, rasping, ringing, wheezing, whistling; from dry cold air; worse from cold water; better from warm food and warm drinks; every mental excitement aggravates cough; worse from talking, singing, smoking.
7. *Orchitis* (inflammation of testicles) : After gonorrhoea or maltreated orchitis.
8. *Aphonia* (voice loss): From exposure to cold (*Acon., Hep., Phos.*).
9. Ailments: with dyspnoea on lying on left side; must lie on right side with head high.
10. Tubercular laryngitis with hoarseness.

## 39. SULPHUR
### (Sulph.)

1. *Diarrhoea*: After midnight; painless; driving out of bed early in the morning; foul smelling; excoriating anus.
2. *Constipation*: Stools hard knotty, dry as if burnt; large; painful.
3. Menorrhagia after miscarriage.
4. Sick headache every week or every two weeks; prostrating; weakening; with hot vertex (top of head) and cold feet.
5. Chronic alcoholism; they reform but are continually relapsing; dropsy and other ailments of drunkards.
6. Third stage of pneumonia when hepatisaton (lung tissue changes into liver-like substance) fails to resolve; aids

resolution of the hepatization of lungs in pneumonia.
7. *Pleurisy:* Pericarditis; helps in the reabsorption of the fluid and plastic exudations, in brain or joints when *Bryonia* fails.
8. *Sulphur* is a specific remedy in the following conditions if the characteristic, constitutional or the anti-miasmatic symptoms are present in the patient: acne; adenoids; alcohol habit; amenorrhoea; asthma; boils; chilblains; constipation; consumption; diarrhoea; dysentery; eczema; eye-affections; haemorrhoids; hypochondriasis; leucorrhoea; liver disorders; lumbago; lupus; measles; menstrual disorders; after-effects of miscarriage; pericarditis; pneumonia; pleurisy; pregnancy disorders; rheumatic disorders; self-abuse; skin affections; sleep disorders (ill-effects of vaccines); startings; urticaria; prolapse of uterus; vaccinosis; worms.
9. **Sulphur should be considered as the remedy in the following conditions:** As a prophylactic remedy in cholera, malaria, recurrent boils; threatening phthisis. As antidote for abuse of metals generally. When syphilis and sycosis are complicated with psora. When partial relief comes from remedies which have no definite complementary remedy. To shorten the convalescent period after acute diseases. When worms are suspected as obstruction to cure. When there is history of suppressed eruptions. When symptoms are left-sided. Should be considered when complaints are relapsing. When exudations are not absorbed. When there is paucity of symptoms. When fever is due to disorder of thermic centre. When the action of other remedies come to a halt. It makes the same remedy work again. When there is in the past history ulcers and other ailments traceable to tuberculosis.
10. **Especially adapted to the following types of patients:**
    (a) children : dirty, filthy; aversion to bath; big belly with emaciated limbs; putting everything in their mouth; watching everyone eating; lips and other orifices of the body are red; restless at night; kicking the covers off even in cold weather; causeless weeping; hungry

yet emaciated; foul odour from perspiration; disposed to skin diseases, worm troubles and excoriating discharges; scrofulous (tubercular) diathesis.

(b) persons of nervous temperament, quick-motioned, quick-tempered, plethoric, skin excessively sensitive to atmospheric changes; lean, thin, hungry, dyspeptic fellow with stooped shoulders, yet many times it must be given to fat, round, well-fed people; persons who lead sedentary life—confined to their rooms in study, in meditation, in philosophical inquiry and who take no exercise—soon find out that they must eat only the simplest food and they end up by going into philosophical mania;

(c) dirty, shrivelled, red-faced people; untidy; not disturbed by uncleanliness; oversensitive to filthy odours but do not hesitate taking filthy substances; with exaggerated sense of smell; discharges are of offensive odour, excoriating the tissues over which they flow; excoriating leucorrhoea, saliva, lachrymation, stools;

(d) patients, who are warm-blooded; complaints come on from becoming warm in bed; burning sensation is found in congestions; burning here and there in spots; burning in the glands, organs, stomach or in lungs, burning stools, urine and discharges; burning of the soles of the feet and palms of hands;

(e) standing is the worst position for *Sulphur* patients; they cannot stand; every standing position is uncomfortable; cramps in calves and soles at night;

(f) *Sulphur* patient is too lazy to rouse himself; too unhappy to live;

(g) *Sulphur* patients are disposed to scrofulous, rachitic, catarrhal, bilious, haemorrhoidal dispositions; tendency to venous and portal (related to pit of a gland for entry of vessels, nerves) congestions; itchy eruptions;

(h) *Sulphur* patients are oxygenoid (needing more oxygen); they suffer from suffocative attacks at night, want the doors and windows open.

11. **Has specific action in the following conditions:**
    (a) when carefully selected remedies fail to produce a favourable effect, especially in acute diseases; it frequently serves to remove the bad effects of psora (itch disease) and rouses the vital reactivity;
    (b) complaints that are continually relapsing due to lack of vital reactivity;
    (c) chronic ailments due to suppressed eruptions causing asthma, epilepsy, chorea, convulsions, diarrhoea, insanity, dyspnoea, vertigo, scrofulous ailments;
    (d) suppression of haemorrhoidal flow causing chronic ailments, including heart troubles;
    (e) chronic ailments from suppressed gonorrhoea, i.e., impotency, prostatic troubles;
    (f) chronic ailments from suppressed eruptions in acute fevers, like small-pox, measles, scarlet fever;
    (g) chronic ailments from suppressed discharges, like menses, sweat, lochia (discharge after delivery);
    (h) drug miasm (poisoning) produced by vaccination.

12. **This remedy should not be given:**
    (a) in advanced cases of pulmonary tuberculosis in high potencies;
    (b) at night to persons who do not suffer from loss of sleep;
    (c) before *Lycopodium*.

## 40. VERATRUM ALBUM
### (Verat.)

1. For ailments with cold sweats on forehead; face pale, blue, collapsed; features sunken, Hippocratic (indicating approach of death); red while lying, becomes pale on rising

up; worse from least motion; great prostration; thirst for large quantities of cold water and acid drinks.

2. *Cholera*: After fright with profuse sweat, profuse vomiting, profuse diarrhoea; thirst for large quantities of cold water; cramps; great prostration; dehydration.

3. *Insanity*: Violent, tears clothes, shrieks, runs about, spits, exposes person, lewd, lascivious talks, sings obscene songs; preaches, talks rapidly, loquacious; praying loudly, religious mania, repents; anxious about salvation, sits brooding, wailing; puerperal insanity, with uterine and menstrual disorders. Catalepsy (trance) from religious excitement. Erotic mania; melancholia; nymphomania (pervetted sexual desire) in lying in women.

4. *Diarrhoea* from fright; fruits; watery, gushing, with cutting colic; with vomiting, cold prespiration on face.

5. Mental troubles from injured pride or honour; disappointed love.

6. Bad effects of opium-eating or tobacco-chewing and alcohol.

7. Shock from injuries with cold sweat on forehead and extreme prostration.

8. Dysmenorrhoea with vomiting and purging.

9. Intermittent fever where cold stage always predominates; with blueness of finger nails; with cold and clammy sweats before the paroxysm begins and lasts until the next.

10. Whooping cough with involuntary urine; vomiting and diarrhoea.

11. Night-blindness preceding menstruation.

12. Vertigo with cold perspiration on head, vomiting and diarrhoea.

13. **Especially adapted to the following types of persons:**
    (a) who are habitually cold;
    (b) who are deficient in vital reaction;

(c) *children*: who are constipated; stools large and hard; when *Nux-v.* and *Lyc.* fail;

(d) young people of a nervous sanguine temperament; inconsolable over fancied misfortune; despair about social position; feel unlucky; want to commit suicide by jumping from a height; brooding, indisposed to talk; sad;

(e) bronchitis of old people with inability to expectorate the large amount of mucus accumulated in the chest;

(f) *hysterical* : thinks she is pregnant, will soon deliver; coldness of body during menstrual periods; anxious and depressed at the time of menses; sensation as if water drunk ran down outside and did not go down the oesophagus (gullet); sensation of a lump of ice on vertex, with chilliness; as if brain is torn to pieces; cannot bear to be left alone yet persistently refuses to talk; attacks of fainting from least exertion; excessive weakness.

## ABOUT MOTHER TINCTURES

**(41) Calendula :** This remedy is used externally and exerts a most favourable influence in promoting the union of wounds with the least resulting scars, and no suppuration. Cuts, whether accidental or inflicted in operations, or injuries, in which the flesh is much torn and which does not heal without the formation of matter or wound cannot be brought together by adhesive plaster, *Calendula* φ is best applied as a wash. Torn wounds should not be handled much. If they bleed, the blood must be stopped as in any other case. If they are dirty, warm water may be gently applied to cleanse them. The wounds should be covered with clean bandage, and kept constantly wet with *Calendula lotion*.

**(42) Cantharis :** As an external remedy, *Cantharis* φ proves efficacious in renal diseases and disorders of mucous membranes. Generally, it prevents blisters formation in cases of accidents by fire, if applied with sufficient promptness. In all cases of burns and scalds, make a lotion—ten drops of the strong tincture to a tea-cupful of water, and sponge the exposed skin night and morning along with the internal administration of *Cantharis* and other remedies for burns and scalds. **Should not be used if the wound is open.**

**(43) Plantago major :** An excellent remedy for local use in toothache in hollow teeth and otorrhoea (pus from ear). For toothache a cotton-wool plug soaked in *Plantago* φ should be kept on the painful teeth to give instant relief from the pain. In case of otorrhoea and otalgia (earache), a drop of *Plantago* φ mixed with a drop of *Mullein oil* may be dipped into the affected ear to get rid of pain and other consequences, with the administration of indicated remedies.

**(44) Mullein oil :** The oil is both sedative and curative in otalgia and otorrhoea and gives best results by using it with *Plantago major* φ.

# 11 | BOOKS RECOMMENDED FOR FURTHER STUDY

| | | |
|---|---|---|
| B. Jain Publishers | : | First Aid Homoeopathy in Accidents & Ailments |
| Bhattacharya, A.K. | : | Family Practice |
| Blackie, M.G. | : | The Patient, Not the Cure |
| Boericke, Garth | : | Homoeopathy |
| Boericke, Garth | : | Principles of Homoeopathy |
| Choudhury, N.M. | : | Study of Materia Medica with Repertory |
| Dewey, W.A. | : | Practical Homoeopathic Therapeutics |
| Gunavante, S.M. | : | Introduction to Homoeopathic Prescribing |
| Hering, C. | : | The Homoeopathic Domestic Physician |
| Hutchinson | : | 700 Redline Symptoms |
| Iyer, T.S. | : | Beginners' Guide to Homoeopathy |
| Jahr, G.H.G. | : | Family Practice with Homoeopathic Remedies |
| Kent, J.T. | : | Lectures on Materia Medica with New Remedies |
| Kent, J.T. | : | Lectures on Homoeopathic Philosophy |
| Krishnamurthy, V. | : | Homoeopathy in Accidents & Injuries |
| Laurie, Joseph | : | An Epitome of the Homoeopathic Domestic Medicine |

| | | |
|---|---|---|
| Mathur, K.N. | : | Guide to Organon |
| Mathur, R.S. | : | Homoeopathy for Layman |
| Pulman Nash | : | Leaders in Homoeopathy |
| Rabe, R.F. | : | Medical Therapeutics for Daily Reference |
| Rawat, P.S. | : | A Self-study course in Homoeopathy |
| Rawat, P.S. | : | Select Your Dose and Potency |
| Ruddock, E.H. | : | Homoeopathic Vade Mecum |
| Ruddock, E.H. | : | The Stepping-stones to Homoeopathy and Health |
| Shinghal, J.N. | : | Quick Bedside Prescriber |
| Singh, Yudhvir | : | Homoeopathic Cure of Common Diseases |
| Smith, A. Dwight | : | The Home Prescriber |
| Smith, A. Dwight | : | Homoeopathy — Rational and Scientific Treatment |
| Smith, Trevor | : | Homoeopathic Medicine |
| Verma, S.P. | : | Clinical Methods |
| Verma, S.P. | : | Guide to Materia Medica |
| Vithoulkas, G. | : | The Science of homoeopathy |
| Vithoulkas, G. | : | The new man of homoeopathy |

A wide range of

books in

Homoeopathy

available at

**B. JAIN PUBLISHERS PVT. LTD.**
1921, Street No. 10th, Chuna Mandi,
Paharganj, New Delhi - 110 055
Tel.: +91-11-4567 1000   Fax: +91-11-4567 1010
Email: info@bjain.com   Website: www.bjain.com